—— PRAISE

GLUTEN-FREE

"Beth Hillson generously shares the w͟ knowledge she has acquired over the many years as a chef, mother, and gluten-free entrepreneur. There are Asian, Jewish, Italian, French, and American favorites. Don't miss the chapter on breads; it's a masterpiece!"

—Rebecca Reilly, author of *Gluten-Free Baking*

"[Hillson's] approach to gluten-free is living with, not living without. Look for alternatives, not at what you can't eat. Be curious, Hillson advises, be imaginative, substitute boldly, and have fun. . . . If you're looking to gain an in-depth understanding of cooking without gluten, *Gluten-Free Makeovers* is an excellent go-to guide and resource to refer back to again and again."

—*San Francisco Book Review*

"Hillson proves that a gluten-free diet doesn't mean that all food choices are taken away."

—*Tucson Citizen*

"This is not your average gluten-free cookbook. It will keep your kitchen humming and you happy with all the treasures you can now produce."

—*Gluten-Free Living*

"These recipe makeovers transform favorite, typically gluten-heavy foods (breads, cakes, pies, pasta, etc.) into safe, appealing options for those with celiac disease, gluten sensitivity, and wheat allergy."

—*Publishers Weekly*

"*Gluten-Free Makeovers* takes you on a culinary journey that's as delicious as it is essential. . . . There's something for every taste—and lots to tempt your taste buds. A must for your kitchen bookshelf."

—*Living Without*

"[Hillson's] recipes were easy to understand and simple to make. . . . This book is great for anyone who lives gluten-free and may not be the best cook in the world."

—*Portland Book Review*

THE COMPLETE GUIDE TO
LIVING WELL
GLUTEN-FREE

THE COMPLETE GUIDE TO

LIVING WELL
GLUTEN-FREE

EVERYTHING YOU NEED TO KNOW TO GO
FROM SURVIVING TO THRIVING

BETH HILLSON

Da Capo
LIFE
LONG

A Member of the Perseus Books Group

Designed by Trish Wilkinson
Set in 11 point Goudy Old Style BT

Library of Congress Cataloging-in-Publication Data

Hillson, Beth.
    The complete guide to living well gluten-free: everything you need to know to go from surviving to thriving / Beth Hillson.
        pages   cm
    Includes bibliographical references and index.
    ISBN 978-0-7382-1708-6 (paperback) — ISBN 978-0-7382-1709-3 (e-book)
1. Gluten-free diet—Popular works. 2. Wheat-free diet—Popular works. 3. Celiac disease—Popular works. 4. Celiac disease—Patients—Life skills guides. I. Title.
RM237.86.H54 2014
641.5'638—dc23   2014015292

First Da Capo Press edition 2014

Published by Da Capo Press
A Member of the Perseus Books Group
www.dacapopress.com

Note: The information in this book is true and complete to the best of our knowledge. This book is intended only as an informative guide for those wishing to know more about health issues. In no way is this book intended to replace, countermand, or conflict with the advice given to you by your own physician. The ultimate decision concerning care should be made between you and your doctor. We strongly recommend you follow his or her advice. Information in this book is general and is offered with no guarantees on the part of the authors or Da Capo Press. The authors and publisher disclaim all liability in connection with the use of this book.

Da Capo Press books are available at special discounts for bulk purchases in the U.S. by corporations, institutions, and other organizations. For more information, please contact the Special Markets Department at the Perseus Books Group, 2300 Chestnut Street, Suite 200, Philadelphia, PA, 19103, or call (800) 810-4145, ext. 5000, or e-mail special. markets@perseusbooks.com.

10 9 8 7 6 5 4 3 2 1

Dedicated to
Joel, Jeremy, and Jennifer
For their love and support

And to my readers
May you always
live well gluten-free

As I see it, every day you do one of two things: build health or produce disease in yourself.

—ADELLE DAVIS, AUTHOR AND NUTRITIONIST (1904–1974)

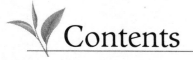

Contents

—— PART ONE ——
The Gluten Question:
Reasons for Adopting a Gluten-free Lifestyle 1

CHAPTER 1

Essential Things You Need to
Know About Celiac Disease   3

—— PART THREE ——

Lifestyle: How to Go from Surviving to Thriving 193

CHAPTER 11

Getting Out: What You Need to Know to Eat and Travel Safely   195

CHAPTER 12

Socializing 225

CHAPTER 13

Friendship, Dating, Love & Sex 261

CHAPTER 14

Coping 275

CHAPTER 15

Living Well: Final Thoughts on a Gluten-free Life Well Lived

Introduction
One Bite at a Time

When I was diagnosed with celiac disease nearly forty years ago, there were no support groups, little information, and few foods. And, oh the food. It tasted like Styrofoam.

I was not motivated to stray from the diet. Gluten made me very sick. Nevertheless, I took little comfort in the pseudo cinnamon buns and slices of bread that reminded me of the toy foods in the Little Tikes kitchen of my childhood. At first it seemed like staying on this diet and eating well were mutually exclusive. But I worked my way back to good health and good food with research, kitchen experiments, and a pledge to create delicious food. My pioneering spirit flourished as I started making baking mixes so I could have freshly baked gluten-free foods whenever I wanted them. As I tasted my first slice of sandwich bread, I knew it was possible to live well again and I wanted to share these great products with others. Soon the Gluten-free Pantry, one of the first gluten-free companies in the United States, was launched.

My customers loved the products, but they also hungered for answers to their questions: Where can I find gluten-free chicken broth? How can I convert my family recipes? How long do I have to wait to have sex after my partner has eaten gluten? And so, along with great food and recipes, I was building a community as I started answering their questions, first in an information newsletter and then in more sophisticated ways. For more than twenty years I have been discussing gluten-free lifestyle issues in weekly newsletters, a twice-weekly blog for Glutino.com, and in blogs and articles for *Gluten Free & More*, formerly *Living Without* magazine, and other publications. And I speak to groups about every aspect of this diet from how to accommodate gluten-free guests to eating safely in restaurants and baking like a pro.

I'm also an advocate for patients and consumers in my role as president of the American Celiac Disease Alliance, a congress made up of leaders from all corners of the gluten-free community. Our shining moment came as we worked with the Food and Drug Administration to establish a gluten-free labeling rule that sets a uniform standard for gluten-free food and makes life safer for those who need a gluten-free diet.

We've come a long way since I was first diagnosed. Store shelves are loaded with gluten-free products and nearly every restaurant offers gluten-free choices. And to think, not long ago physicians were reluctant to put people on the gluten-free diet, believing it was a horrible life sentence. How times have changed.

Today, millions of people freely choose *gluten-free* over *gluten-filled* and physicians are quick to suggest a gluten-free diet for a wide range of ailments. It's a popular diet, even trendy, thanks to a growing number of best-selling books on the problems with gluten and testimonials by celebrities and athletes who tout the benefits of a life without gluten. This trend translates into a multibillion-dollar industry and a supporting cast of thousands of assorted health professionals, natural food authorities, writers, and bloggers.

While there is more information than anyone can digest these days, myths and misinformation abound, too. So, how can you tell what's safe and what's not? Whatever the reason you come to this diet, I'll help you sort through the maze.

Perhaps you've been diagnosed with celiac disease, nonceliac gluten-sensitivity, or a wheat allergy. Or maybe you feel bloated when you eat gluten and want to give the gluten-free diet a try. And, whether you avoid gluten for a serious medical reason or because you feel better, I hear you when you say you're riding an emotional roller coaster. One day, you feel great because you've made delicious bread without gluten; the next, you are having a meltdown because Thanksgiving is coming, you don't want to stray from the diet, but the menu seems impossible to navigate. One moment, you are managing all the tasks in your gluten-free checklist (going to follow-up doctor visits, checking vitamin levels, stocking extra rolls for lunches); and the next, it seems impossible to keep track of all these new layers of life. When children are involved, it's even more complicated. Gluten creeps into every aspect of life. I know. Since my son, Jeremy, and my sister, Jennifer, also have celiac disease, this is not a lifestyle I treat lightly.

Whether your reason is medical or it just seems like a healthier lifestyle, this book helps you navigate gluten-free living with aplomb. It's aimed at fortifying you with knowledge and coping skills. In essence, it's the book I wish I had when I was diagnosed forty years ago, a book to help you live well gluten-free.

Besides a wealth of information, it is filled with encouragement, support, and personal stories (see Gut Reactions). By sharing my own experiences, I put a human face on this challenging lifestyle. If I am willing to discuss my own condition, I am hoping you will feel more comfortable embracing yours.

I'm not a medical professional, but as you know if you've already tried a gluten-free diet, a diagnosis or decision to go gluten-free is just the beginning of this journey.

So take a deep breath, smile, and follow me as I answer all your questions and shed some light on things you didn't even know to ask. You can do this; just take it one bite at a time.

About This Book

I remember the loneliness that washed over me when I was diagnosed with celiac disease and was told I could not eat anything with gluten. I was overwhelmed imagining how I would manage. The prospect of a breadless future was not appetizing. My doctor handed me two pages of resources to help. It was everything anyone knew about the gluten-free diet. Imagine. The entire blueprint for my new, gluten-free life was summed up in two pages!

It's a new world chock-full of information and food choices.

There's a lot to tell and this fascinating topic changes by the minute.

- While I was writing the book, the gluten-free labeling rule was released. This clears the air on confusing labels that say "made in a facility that also uses wheat." Now consumers know when a product label says "gluten-free" it has to have less than 20 parts per million of gluten. (I'll explain what *parts per million* means in Chapter 6.)
- New treatments to supplement the gluten-free diet (or cure celiac disease) are on the horizon and may mean we'll have a pill or a vaccine in the next decade.
- Work is under way to develop biomarkers for gluten sensitivity, and with it, the capability of diagnosing this elusive condition and predicting the size of the gluten-sensitive population.

- Nearly 90 million Americans, or about 29 percent, are eating gluten-free at least some of the time.
- Whether you are gluten-free for medical reasons or by choice, the challenges of managing this diet are the same.

But I discovered a few surprises, too:

- Many physicians are still not aware of the hereditary component of celiac disease and that all first-degree relatives should be tested.
- A food product label saying "contains no gluten ingredients," but not saying "gluten-free" on the package does not have to comply with the less than 20 ppm threshold of gluten set out in the new gluten-free food labeling regulation. (If this is Greek to you, we'll make sense of labeling on pages 118–125.)

This is just the tip of the proverbial gluten-free iceberg! In this book you'll find detailed info covering every aspect of the gluten-free life, from diagnosis to kitchen basics (yours and someone else's) to lifestyle questions, travel, kids, even managing a child's diet in a divorce—everything you need to know to thrive. Here are some of the topics I tackle:

- What's the difference between gluten sensitivity and celiac disease
- When is it safe to kiss your date who has been eating gluten
- The best age to introduce your baby to gluten
- What to do if an insurance company turns you down for a preexisting condition
- How to set up a school lunch program for your child
- How to talk to a restaurant chef to determine his or her understanding of your diet

There are also sections called "Raising Your Gluten-free IQ." They set the record straight on myths and misinformation and present some facts that might surprise you. For instance, can you believe a friend who tells you heat removes gluten, a doctor who says she ruled out celiac disease by performing a colonoscopy, a nutritionist who says he has a test for gluten sensitivity? While all this may seem overwhelming, it's what you'll need to know to stay well and healthy.

And perhaps you are here because you suspect you have an intolerance to gluten or an allergy or you've heard about the health benefits of a gluten-free diet. This book will answer your questions and get you headed in the right direction, too.

Trust Your Gut:
The Last Word Is YOURS

Use this material as a place to start, not the final word. It's meant to guide you into a lifestyle that works for you and has worked for me. Don't worry about making every day a perfectly gluten-free day. Just try your best and don't cheat intentionally.

Once you've read a section that is helpful, you might put the book aside for a while. Then begin incorporating tips into your lifestyle. Or you might thumb through sections over and over.

Whatever works for you is the right approach. And don't do anything unless or until it feels right. Trust your gut.

Disclaimer

The information in this book is meant to be a guideline—friendly advice from a seasoned traveler in the gluten-free world. But it is not meant to serve as medical advice. You need to get that from your own physician, someone who knows your personal history. I suggest taking this information or the names of research papers mentioned here when you visit your doctor and let it be a place to start a discussion that will lead you on the road to good health.

In addition, ingredients and food products are often reformulated. Read labels every time you purchase a product to be sure it is still safe for your diet.

Gluten Tag: Say Hello to a New Gluten-free Day

When my son, Jeremy, came home for the Christmas holiday in 2012, he found me fretting between turkey and titles. I had written several possible names for this book and the list was taped to the refrigerator. As I washed salad, measured ingredients for my gluten-free bread, and stuffed my turkey, I walked around the kitchen reciting each contender. Nothing worked.

Then one dark and stormy night, he and several friends gathered in my kitchen, fortified to stave off the gloom with a bottle of Scotch, a plate of tacos, several ballpoint pens, and a generous helping of wit.

In the morning, the Scotch and the tacos were gone. The pens were strewn across the counter. And the paper on the refrigerator was covered in sprawling letters, each line a new, hilarious contender.

- No Gluten, No Tootin'
- Vladimir Gluten: Guide to GF Russian Cuisine
- Gluten Tag! Say Hello to a New Gluten-free Day
- The Last of the Gluhicans
- The Anguish of Change: Gluten and the Fall of Man
- Encyclopedia Glutenica
- Fifty Shades of Diarrhea

I stood in front of the refrigerator with mug in hand and roared until the coffee splashed over the top of my cup. Their humor and ideas spilled off that sheet and onto this project. But I kept a good helping bottled by my desk. No, it's not Scotch, but it is intoxicating. There is no substitute for hearty laughter. It's good stuff. It's free and it's gluten-free. I recommend a daily dose.

The Faces of Gluten-free
Who Needs This Diet

There are so many reasons that people avoid gluten, these days. I don't think there are enough pages here to give you all a face. First, let's look at the medical reasons that someone needs a gluten-free diet.

Perhaps you've been diagnosed with an autoimmune condition, such as celiac disease, dermatitis herpetiformis, or gluten ataxia. This group comprises about 1 percent of Americans—people with an autoimmune disease that is diagnosed by means of blood tests and/or small bowel biopsy and genetic markers. For this group, the gluten-free diet is a medical necessity. (Dermatitis herpetiformis and gluten ataxia affect a small percentage of this group and while the gluten-free diet is the mandatory treatment, the diagnosis will include some additional tests. We'll talk about these conditions in the Diagnosis portion of this book.)

Physicians refer to people with celiac disease as celiac patients or people with celiac disease. I don't like to call people celiacs as it implies that they are defined by the illness. It is self-limiting. Nonetheless, I sometimes slip and refer to those of us with celiac disease simply as celiacs. My apologies. I don't mean to offend anyone. But it slips into conversation from time to time. In your mind, please know that the word *patient* is always there, but sometimes it's silent.

Still another group comes to this diet because even though they don't test positive for celiac disease, gluten makes them very sick. They are the folks with nonceliac gluten sensitivity. The diagnosis is made by exclusion. Although they test negative for other gluten-related illnesses, such as celiac disease and wheat allergy, the only way to alleviate symptoms is to eliminate gluten. We used to call this gluten intolerance. Now it has its own name and medical description.

Some medical researchers believe the number of people who have nonceliac gluten sensitivity may be much larger than the celiac population (3 to 6 percent of Americans). Others suggest that it's closer to 1 percent. At this point, we are not even sure the culprit is just gluten. (We'll talk about this, too.)

While the correct terminology for this category is "nonceliac gluten sensitivity," for purposes of this book, I sometimes refer to it as simply "gluten sensitive." The "nonceliac" part is silent. Those who have it know who they are.

A small number have a wheat allergy, and as wheat is a large component of the gluten-free diet, they will find help in this gluten-free book as well. Immune rather than autoimmune, wheat allergy is also a medical diagnosis.

Then there's the largest group. These people have given up gluten by choice rather than because of a medical necessity. I can't begin to put a face on all the reasons they've chosen this regimen. Some may fall into one of the other categories and chose the route of self-diagnosis. Perhaps they've read a best-selling book that makes a compelling argument for giving up gluten. Or maybe their physical therapist suggested that a gluten-free diet might reduce the inflammation in their knee. Some practitioners tie gluten to high blood sugar; others report that genetically modified wheat is bad for all of us. (For the record, scientists tell us that wheat is not genetically modified.) Maybe one of these folks struck a chord. Whether it's to lose weight, curb heart disease, stop dementia, or as a pathway to overall better health, those who belong to this group know why they've decided to give up gluten. All together, the "gluten-free by choice," group represents up to 29 percent of the population and it's growing. (In this book, I refer to this group as gluten avoiders, too.)

It's not for me to say whether you should or should not give up gluten. But I do know that anecdotal symptoms can be just as real as those of someone who has gluten sensitivity or celiac disease. Whatever your reason, I want you to be healthy, feel good, and navigate this diet with skill and comfort. You'll find all the important ingredients to do so in the pages of this book.

The Numbers Game: Just Who Is Eating Gluten-free?

If you are on a gluten-free diet or thinking about going gluten-free, join the club, a very large club, indeed. Millions of Americans have taken up the gluten-free regimen.

We know from a large study published by Alessio Fasano, MD, at the Center for Celiac Research in 2003, that about 3 million have celiac disease. We also know that most (about 80 to 85 percent) are yet to be diagnosed. Where did all these other gluten-free folks come from?

People with nonceliac gluten sensitivity make up a portion of that group. Some researchers estimate that between 3 and 6 percent of the US population has a sensitivity to gluten that is not celiac disease. And, based on market research, it's estimated that an additional 23 to 29 percent of the American population has adopted a gluten-free lifestyle because of health concerns, other disorders, or the perception that eating gluten-free food is a healthier lifestyle. If my calculations are correct, that means around 90 million people are avoiding gluten at least part of the time.

Nevertheless, celiac disease remains at the center of this much larger population of gluten-free consumers. If people switch their allegiance to another way of eating or research finds that gluten sensitivity is triggered by something other than gluten, this core of nearly 3 million people will still need a gluten-free diet.

Terms and Acronyms

Terms

Allergy: An allergy is an immune response to something that appears harmful outside the body. It can be outgrown.

Asymptomatic celiac disease: Celiac disease patients who have positive antibodies and genetic tests but do not present with symptoms usually associated with the disease. These folks should still follow a gluten-free diet.

Autoimmune disease: When the body attacks itself, harming healthy body tissue rather than attacking a foreign substance. An autoimmune disorder cannot be outgrown. It's for life.

Celiac disease: An autoimmune disease triggered by ingestion of gluten, the protein in wheat, rye, and barley. It is diagnosed by positive antibody tests, genetic markers, and intestinal damage shown on biopsy.

Cross-contamination and cross-contact: These terms are synonymous when discussed in relation to the gluten-free diet. Both refer to gluten-free food coming in contact with gluten-containing foods because they are processed in a shared space.

Gluten: Gluten is an amino acid sequence found in wheat, rye, and barley. It's not one substance; rather, a complex structure of peptides or prolamins that are broken down into gliadins and glutenins. The gliadins are thought to be the primary cause of celiac disease, but some patients react to other proteins in this sequence as well.

Gluten gives elasticity to dough, helping it rise and keep its shape. Gluten-free bakers are on a never-ending quest to discover suitable substitutes for wheat and gluten in baked foods.

Gluten allergy: This is not really a medical term. You are allergic to individual grains, not gluten. People who cannot have gluten, including those with celiac disease, dermatitis herpetiformis, gluten ataxia, and nonceliac gluten sensitivity, may say they are allergic to gluten because "allergy" is easier to explain than celiac disease. This is different than wheat allergy (see page xxxiv), which is a specific allergy to components of wheat and includes specific tests.

Gluten-ed by proxy: When you entrust another person to manage your diet and assume he or she knows it as well as you do, your chance of getting gluten-ed goes up by a factor of that person's lack of knowledge and education about gluten. On page 255 we discuss ways to minimize that risk. But for now, remember that if you assume that someone understands your diet as well as you do, you stand a chance of being gluten-ed by proxy.

Gluten-free by choice (a.k.a. gluten avoiders): Those who follow a gluten-free diet as a personal preference and lifestyle choice.

Gluten-free diet (GFD): A diet free of all wheat, rye, and barley.

Gluten-free friendly (GFF): People or places that have some familiarity with the gluten-free diet and a willingness to help gluten-free people eat safely.

Gluten-free oats: The form of gluten in pure oats (not contaminated with wheat) is a different protein than that found in wheat, rye, and barley and safe for a gluten-free diet. But for many years, people with celiac disease were told to avoid them probably because most oats are grown in fields and/or processed on shared equipment with wheat. Oats that are labeled "gluten-free" are grown using methods that eliminate this cross-contamination and test at less than 20 parts per million of gluten. Nevertheless, some people with celiac disease and gluten sensitivity cannot eat these oats, either.

Gluten-related disorders or gluten spectrum disorders: You'll hear this term from time to time. It's a broad group of disorders related to ingesting gluten. This includes several conditions, including celiac disease, dermatitis herpetiformis, gluten ataxia, and nonceliac gluten sensitivity. While these all fit under one umbrella, according to a medical paper from 2012, they each have a specific diagnosis. At the moment, nonceliac gluten sensitivity is diagnosed by the exclusion of celiac disease, and gluten ataxia is often diagnosed by exclusion, too.

Gluten smooching: When a gluten-free person is kissed by someone who has just eaten a lot of gluten.

- Your baby reaches up for a smooch, shoving his little hands into your mouth. Only he's just eaten animal crackers or Cheerios and his face and hands are covered with gluten.
- You bend down to kiss your dog that has just eaten dog food containing gluten.
- You are on a first date and have not had "The Talk" about gluten with your companion. After downing a pizza and a cold beer, he (or she) enthusiastically plants a big one on your lips.

Latent celiac disease: Latent celiac disease is when a person tests positive for one celiac antibody but has no intestinal damage when a biopsy is done. If you are told you have latent celiac disease, this means you are at risk for developing the disease and should be monitored regularly by your doctor. Another confusing diagnosis is silent celiac disease (see page xxxiv), and they are not the same.

Nontropical sprue: Also known as celiac sprue, this is the name once used for celiac disease.

Potential celiac disease: A person who has a positive antibody test for celiac disease but a normal biopsy of the small intestine is considered at risk for developing celiac disease. Doctors recommend close follow-up of these patients.

Sensitivity versus allergy: Medically, these terms are not synonymous and are treated differently, but we lay folks often use them interchangeably. When I am speaking to a server in a restaurant or a casual acquaintance,

I am likely to say I'm allergic to gluten. It's not true. But to tell people I have an autoimmune disease or a sensitivity seems like too much information. I don't think they want to know all the details.

Mostly we just want to get the message across that we will get pretty sick if we eat gluten and might just crap our pants right in the restaurant. Sometimes that trumps technicalities.

In the Diagnosis section of this book, we talk about the medical terminology. If you slip and call it an allergy when you mean sensitivity or celiac, it's okay with me. Your doctor will be far more specific, as he or she should be.

Seriously gluten-free: This lay term is often used by people in the restaurant industry to differentiate people who will become ill if they ingest even tiny amounts of gluten from those who simply avoid gluten ingredients.

Silent celiac disease: Silent celiac disease is when you have no symptoms but test positive for antibodies and a small intestine biopsy is positive. Many people with celiac disease have no outward symptoms. Often the doctor tests you because of a secondary issue that is not improving, such as osteoporosis, infertility, or unexplained anemia. People in this group must adhere to a gluten-free diet.

Subclinical celiac disease: Unsuspected celiac disease. The patient has no symptoms or signs that would prompt a physician to test them. The diagnosis is often made by "accident" when a physician is trying to find the cause of anemia, osteoporosis, or acid reflux, for instance.

Wheat allergy: An immune response to wheat ingestion. Symptoms can be sniffling, itching, hives, difficulty breathing, and swelling of the throat and airway. Wheat allergy can also lead to cramps, nausea, and vomiting. The symptoms can appear within minutes or a few hours after eating wheat. In extreme cases, it can be life-threatening. The body is reacting to one of several proteins in wheat, including gluten, but this is not the same as celiac or gluten sensitivity (think: immune rather than autoimmune). Most people who have a wheat allergy can eat barley, rye, and oats as well as some forms of wheat, such as spelt, einkorn, kamut, and farro. It's more common in children than in adults and can be outgrown.

Acronyms

FALCPA: Food Allergen Labeling and Consumer Protection Act of 2004, regulated by the US Food and Drug Administration (FDA) and mandating that all food products must list any of the eight top food allergens contained in the product (eggs, fish, milk, peanuts, shellfish, soy, tree nuts, wheat). This is a label of exclusion. If a food label says "contains wheat," it's not safe for a gluten-free diet.

FDA: US Food and Drug Administration, the government organization responsible for issuing and overseeing the gluten-free labeling regulations on food products except meats and poultry (regulated by the US Department of Agriculture [USDA]) and alcohol (regulated by the Tax and Trade Bureau [TTB]). This is a label of inclusion. Products labeled "gluten-free" are safe for a gluten-free diet.

GF: Gluten-free

GFD: Gluten-free diet

PPM: Parts per million. For purposes of this book, it relates to the level of gluten medically determined to be safe for most people with celiac disease (less than 20 ppm).

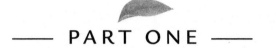

— PART ONE —

The Gluten Question

Reasons for Adopting a
Gluten-free Lifestyle

Does it seem to you that the whole world is on a gluten-free diet (GFD) these days? No surprise. At least one market research group says nearly 30 percent of Americans are choosing gluten-free over gluten-filled food.

If you are one of them, you are certainly not alone. People come to the regimen for a hundred reasons. Perhaps you've read a bestselling book that makes a compelling case for the benefits of a life without gluten. Maybe you've heard television celebrities tout the benefits of giving up gluten to drop some weight. Or a physical therapist suggested the diet to reduce joint pain or reduce inflammation in a shoulder. And a smaller number of you have been diagnosed with celiac disease, related autoimmune conditions, or gluten sensitivity. For you (and me), the GFD is a medical imperative. We'll be on this diet for life.

Whether you are here because of a medical diagnosis, an alternative diet regimen, or a lifestyle decision, this part will help you sort out the various gluten-related conditions, tests, and diagnoses; talk about other reasons people might give up gluten; and ultimately help you take the best step forward.

Essential Things You Need to Know About Celiac Disease

We're going to cover a lot of info in this chapter, so get your highlighter ready. First things first: if you suspect that you have a gluten-related illness . . .

You Need to Rule Out Celiac Disease Before Going Gluten-free

Chew on this for a moment. You adopt a gluten-free diet. A light goes off when you notice you feel better, have less gas, fewer digestion issues, more energy. "Maybe I have celiac disease," you might say. "I think I should be tested."

Feeling better is great news. But here's the bad news. *You can't be tested for celiac disease unless you are eating gluten.* Your body only makes the antibodies to gluten if you eat it. So, before you go gluten-free, do yourself a favor and get tested for celiac disease. Once you're feeling good, do you want to go through eating gluten again?

That's what I thought.

Additionally, you need to rule out celiac disease before you can be diagnosed with nonceliac gluten sensitivity.

Why You Should Be Tested

After falling through the cracks of the medical system, I wonder how many people become frustrated and give up on diagnosis, choosing to adopt a gluten-free lifestyle without further testing. Adopting this regimen can be a challenge at times, but now it's easier than ever before; information on the diet and so many good food choices abound. And the bonus: you feel better.

How many who have fallen through the medical hierarchy actually have celiac disease? If, after years of suffering and getting nowhere with traditional medicine, you feel better on a gluten-free diet, who's to say you shouldn't go gluten-free? Or perhaps instead of testing you, your doctor suggested you give the GFD a try. Horror of horrors. Because this diet is so popular, many health professionals are recommending it. "If it was diabetes, you wouldn't suggest trying a little insulin without testing the patient," says Alice Bast, president of the National Foundation for Celiac Awareness (NFCA). She makes a good point.

Maybe that is why you are here now—reading this book! But, aside from not being able to get a diagnosis (or ruling it out) if you aren't eating gluten, there are many more reasons that you need to know whether you have celiac disease:

- Celiac disease is an autoimmune disease that can affect every system in your body and lead to other conditions. If you get sick, your doctor will be better informed if he or she knows you have celiac disease.
- You need to know how strict you need to be with the diet. Tiny amounts of gluten can still cause gut damage and other long-term health effects if you're celiac; not so if you are gluten sensitive or avoid gluten by choice.
- Celiac disease is hereditary; first-degree relatives (that means parents, siblings, and children) of a celiac patient should be tested.
- Under the Americans with Disabilities Act, students with celiac disease may qualify for gluten-free school lunches.
- Children with celiac disease may be growing poorly or have behavioral or learning issues affecting schoolwork and the ability to social-

ize. Wouldn't it be amazing if the diagnosis of celiac disease and a GFD was all it took to avoid having your kid "labeled" in school?

- If you have celiac disease and are trying to have a baby but not sticking to a 100 percent gluten-free diet, staying true to the diet might help you get pregnant.
- If you are pregnant and not following the diet all the time, it can lead to miscarriage or low-birth-weight children.
- Living with undiagnosed celiac disease can shorten your life expectancy. There is a higher incidence of intestinal cancers, lymphoma, and even hip fractures related to untreated celiac disease.
- You can take a deduction for the cost of your gluten-free food on your income taxes—but only if you've been officially diagnosed.
- Relief from your symptoms (think: bloating, gas, and fatigue) can improve your sex life, give you more energy and more desire. And who doesn't want more satisfying sex?
- Now here's the big one. You can't be counted among celiac patients unless you are diagnosed, and numbers matter. Why do you need to be counted? There are a number of reasons, but two of the important ones are better insurance coverage and more research dollars. You need only look at the prevalence studies on page 7 and the history that led up to this research, and you'll understand that no one was studying celiac disease when it was considered very rare.

Do the Math: Prevalence of Celiac Disease

One of the chief reasons that the medical community has been slow to make the celiac diagnosis in patients is that physicians are still unaware the disease is so prevalent.

In 1993 (when I founded one of the first gluten-free companies in the United States, the Gluten-free Pantry), the number of people with celiac disease was thought to be 1 in 1,000.

Around the year 2000, one of the leading physicians in the celiac medical community, Dr. Alessio Fasano, began suggesting that the number of celiac patients was higher than we believed, more like 1 in 100, the prevalence in Italy where he had received his medical degree at the prestigious

Gut Reaction: It's Relative

For years I thought I was the only one in my family with celiac disease. But in 1993 my son (then age six) was diagnosed.

My sister got the surprising diagnosis in 2005, after being diagnosed with severe osteoporosis. Although she is very active and seemingly healthy, she could not boost her blood calcium level, no matter how hard she tried. Then the doctor prescribed Actonel, a strong medication that is used to help increase bone density. That made matters worse. Because she was not absorbing calcium, the Actonel was drawing it from her bones, decreasing her bone density even further.

To step back for a moment, in 2001, I had marched all my first-degree relatives to our local support group to be tested for celiac disease as part of a blood screening conducted by Dr. Alessio Fasano, one of the leading physicians in the celiac medical community. The test was the most advanced and the most sensitive. Everyone in my family, including my sister, tested negative. Looking back, it's likely she (and maybe others) is deficient in the antibody that makes that particular form of the test reliable, giving her a false negative result (for more information on these tests and how they work, see Chapter 3).

We were surprised, then, when an endoscopy in 2005 showed that my sister's villi were damaged, proof positive for celiac disease. After she had been on a gluten-free diet for six months, I asked her whether she noticed any difference. She said she no longer had a "nervous stomach" or the sudden urges to rush to the bathroom after meals. How long had she had those symptoms? "Since I was fifteen," she replied. She was fifty-two when she was diagnosed.

My son and I count ourselves among the lucky ones. We were diagnosed as children. Research shows that early diagnosis reduces the possibility of having other related health issues, including osteoporosis, lymphomas, and other autoimmune diseases, such as Hashimoto's disease. Fortunately, the awareness both in the general public and the medical community has grown dramatically in the last decade. You are among the fortunate ones if you are diagnosed, these days. You can trade crappy and cranky for happy, thankful, and healthy.

University of Naples. A multicenter study on the prevalence of celiac disease in the United States was published by Dr. Fasano in February 2003 and it showed that celiac disease affects about 1 in 133 people, or an estimated 3 million Americans.[1]

Dr. Fasano's study also revealed a significant hereditary component to celiac disease. In people with a first-degree relative (parent, child, sibling) who has celiac disease, the occurrence is 1 in 22; and it's 1 in 39 for people with a second-degree relative (aunt, uncle, cousin) who has the disease. The study also found that only 35 percent of patients diagnosed during the study had chronic diarrhea, and 60 percent of children and 41 percent of adults diagnosed during the study had no symptoms.

This landmark study marked a turning point in the field of celiac disease and a life-changer for diagnosed patients like my son and me. Celiac disease was no longer to be viewed as something rare, said the leading researchers. Physicians became more aware of the disease and began screening for it through blood work.

Note: You'll see this number, too: According to the National Health and Nutrition Examination Survey (NHANES), 2009–2010, the prevalence of celiac disease is 1 in 141. However, this survey excluded children under the age of six.[2]

The Symptoms:
Celiac Disease—the Great Impersonator

Celiac disease is the great imitator. It has lots of things going on and the symptoms can be confused with so many other conditions. You have to put it together.

—ROBERT G. SCHWARTZ, MD, GASTROENTEROLOGIST

Celiac disease is an autoimmune disease. While it expresses itself in the small intestine when gluten is eaten, the disease can affect other systems in the body as well. Although there is a marked increase in those diagnosed with celiac disease, surprisingly most people with celiac disease are thought to be undiagnosed or misdiagnosed. According to the University of Chicago Celiac Disease Center, 85 percent of those with celiac disease don't know it! Other leading experts say the number of undiagnosed patients is between 82 and 90 percent. Since this is not a reportable condition, no one knows for sure. Only 30 percent of adult celiac patients have textbook symptoms, such as bloating, gas, diarrhea, weight loss, and digestive upset. That means a full 70 percent have nonspecific symptoms or no symptoms at all. Often the diagnosis is made when the patient has another ailment (such as anemia, infertility, eczema, or osteoporosis) that cannot be explained and doesn't respond to normal treatment.

Although doctor awareness and diagnostic tools are much better than they were even five years ago, it is still a difficult disease to diagnose, as it masquerades in a host of other conditions from the very subtle, such as acid reflux, to the more specific, such as osteoporosis, tooth enamel defects, central and peripheral nervous system disease, pancreatic disease, internal hemorrhaging, organ disorders (gall bladder, liver, and spleen), and gynecological disorders, including infertility.

Untreated celiac disease has also been linked to an increased risk of certain types of cancer, particularly intestinal lymphoma and bowel cancer, and recent studies have shown an increase in hip fractures, too. In total, celiac disease is associated with approximately two hundred symptoms, according to the University of Chicago Celiac Disease Center.

No matter what kinds of symptoms or severity of symptoms you experience when you eat gluten, untreated celiac disease can be life-threatening.

Here are some of the most common symptoms:[3]

- Frequent abdominal bloating and pain
- Chronic diarrhea or constipation
- Vomiting
- Heartburn
- Weight loss
- Pale, foul-smelling stool
- Iron-deficiency anemia that does not respond to iron therapy
- Fatigue
- Failure to thrive or short stature

- Delayed puberty
- Pain in the joints
- Tingling or numbness in the legs (neuropathy)
- Pale sores inside the mouth
- A skin rash called dermatitis herpetiformis
- Tooth discoloration or loss of enamel
- Unexplained infertility or recurrent miscarriage
- Osteopenia (mild) or osteoporosis (more serious bone density problem)
- Peripheral neuropathy (nerve damage)
- Mental health disorders, such as anxiety or depression

Celiac Disease and Malnutrition

Celiac disease is sometimes referred to as malabsorption syndrome. A person with undiagnosed celiac disease can eat amazing amounts of food and still virtually starve to death. Here's why.

The exact cause of celiac disease is unknown. But we know it affects the mucosal lining of the small intestine, damaging the fingerlike projections called villi.

Remember high school biology? Adults have about 25 feet of small intestine. Between 3 and 7 million wavy, hairlike projections, the villi, line the intestinal wall. Together they are the area of two football fields.

The villi are the workhorses of our digestive system. This is the place where most of our nutrients, vitamins, and minerals are absorbed and sent happily into the bloodstream to fuel the other parts of our body. That is, unless we have celiac disease.

When people with celiac disease eat foods containing gluten, the immune system reacts as if the gluten is an infection and rushes to attack it. As this battle rages, the villi are damaged, inflamed, and worn away. Whether the patient has symptoms or not, this takes place continually as long as gluten is eaten. The damage impairs the ability to absorb nutrients. When the gut is damaged, no matter how much food is eaten, the patient becomes malnourished and seriously deficient in many vitamins, including B_{12}, B_6, and D, as well as iron, calcium, folic acid, niacin, copper, riboflavin, carnitine, and zinc. Many of us heard stories of relatives from the past who just *wasted away*. How many do you suppose had undiagnosed celiac disease?

Note: Although every patient presents with different symptoms, villous atrophy must be present to make the diagnosis of celiac disease.

Intake and Output: The Poop on Poop

Everyone poops. But the quality of that poop is what sets us apart. Here's a discreet tidbit on this delicate subject. People with digestive diseases, such as celiac, or gluten sensitivity (irritable bowel syndrome or colitis, too) are fixated on their bathroom habits. And for good reason.

People whose villi are worn away and whose intestinal lining is irritated can suffer endless bouts of diarrhea so severe they cannot leave the house. Others are bound with severe constipation. No amount of laxative can break the cycle.

We go through endless mental exercises trying to figure out what we ate or drank and what might be causing these discomforts and there's plenty of time to reflect on previous meals while we sit in the bathroom.

Once a diagnosis and diet have been prescribed, we begin to feel better and our symptoms subside. But we watch and wait and worry that debilitating symptoms will return. And the way to check? You guessed it. The formation of the poop. A little loose, a bit gassy, too big, too firm—and we reflect back two days, or two hours, and ask, "What did I eat?"

A note about gluten sensitivity: We'll talk more about gluten sensitivity in Chapter 3, but it's worth mentioning now that while gluten-sensitive people do not have the damage to the small intestine, they are not free from these discomforts. In fact, diarrhea or constipation might be their only symptom.

Dial *D* for Diarrhea

When I owned Gluten-free Pantry, it was not unusual for a customer service representative to spend hours on the phone, discussing intimate issues with a customer: Was it normal to poop three to six times a day? How long do I need to wait before having sex if my partner has eaten gluten? What do I do if my husband (or ex) allows my child to cheat on the diet? Some of these questions went beyond the job description. So, when we added a fancy phone system, we considered adding extensions for people who just wanted to talk about poop. Part of the message would be: *Press D for diarrhea; C for constipation, for all other calls please hold for the next available person, who might be in the bathroom.*

Gut Reaction: I Could Have Been the Poster Child

You could say I was a poster child for celiac disease. When I was diagnosed the first time in the early fifties, I was a small child and celiac disease was considered a childhood disease with textbook symptoms: large, foul-smelling stool, failure to thrive, and a distended belly.

We now know this classic presentation is only the tip of the proverbial celiac iceberg. People present at all ages and with classic or atypical symptoms or none at all.

Back then, the disease was considered rare because few people had been diagnosed, and because the screening and diagnosis were difficult. Who would put their kid through that invasive procedure unless it was essential?

In my case, I complained that my tummy hurt. My belly protruded beyond a slender frame and my bowel movements plugged the toilet on a regular basis. "How could a little kid poop so much?" my father often asked. These symptoms got the attention of my parents and my pediatrician who feared I had cystic fibrosis. So off we went to Boston Children's Hospital to rule out that horrible disease.

At Children's, a sea of nurses and doctors stuck endless tubes into my mouth and nose and needles into my fingers to take blood. (For the record, I was not a good patient.) One of the tests meant swallowing a flexible tube called a Crosby capsule and letting the bulb at my end find its way to the right spot in the small intestine. The doctor then pushed a plunger at his end and, if all went well, harvested a snippet of intestinal lining. It took several hours and intermittent fluoroscopy before the tube reached the correct location.

▶

▼

My parents were grateful when the biopsy confirmed nontropical sprue (the old name for celiac disease) instead of cystic fibrosis. I was grateful to get out of the hospital, get home, and tell my friends that I was a *silly act*.

Nearly everything edible was taken away, and for months I lived on bananas, an awful soy milk formula, and heaping tablespoons of greenish-yellow vitamin B syrup. I was, indeed, one of the proverbial banana babies.

Ironically, the word *gluten* was never mentioned. Foods were added back one by one until, nearly four years later, I was able to have starches and sugar—corn, potatoes, sugar, peas, and finally wheat. And then I was *cured** and could return to eating a normal diet.

Just as large stools had been the hallmark of my symptoms, good poops were the trademark of my *cure*. As new foods were added, my mother was instructed to notice any changes in my bathroom habits before she added another new food.

If they feel like sharing, anyone who's been diagnosed with celiac disease or gluten sensitivity will tell you that we are bathroom people, fixated on our toilet habits, monitoring for signs of ill health or good health. Life with celiac disease or gluten sensitivity is an ongoing process of intake and output.

---

*Of course, today, we know that gluten is the culprit and there is no cure for celiac disease, no medication, just a 100 percent gluten-free diet for life.

Dental Enamel Defects and Celiac Disease

Tooth enamel defects are another fairly common symptom of celiac disease, most often associated with children. I'm talking about tooth discoloration, poor enamel formation, pitting or banding on the teeth, or mottled or translucent-looking teeth. There are other causes for tooth enamel issues, too, such as fluoride treatments or if the mother took tetracycline during pregnancy, so this is not always an indication of celiac disease. Nevertheless, if your dentist notices something weird in the way your child's teeth are forming, this might be a reason to test your child for celiac disease. The dental defects can be treated cosmetically, but the condition will not improve once you remove gluten.

Depression, Anxiety, and Other Mental Health Issues

The brain-body relationship can't be overlooked. Although medically a connection between celiac disease and mental health is not well documented, we all know we function better when we eat well. Many undiagnosed celiac patients are not having those positive feelings. In fact, they report a lack of well-being that includes depression and anxiety.

By itself, a clinical diagnosis for depression and anxiety is hard to make. Couple that with a patient who goes to the doctor complaining of persistent, nonspecific symptoms, such as vague tummy issues, indigestion, difficulty sleeping, or irritability, and it's not unusual for a physician to overlook the possibility of celiac disease and suggest psychiatric care or antidepressants instead.

But we know that celiac patients are often deficient in several key vitamins, such as folate (folic acid), and vitamins B_{12} and B_6, which are related to well-being. Absorbed in the upper portion of the small intestine (the duodenum), a deficiency of folate is shown to increase irritability and forgetfulness, according to Peter H. R. Green, MD, and Rory Jones in *Celiac Disease: A Hidden Epidemic*.[4] In addition, low levels of vitamins B_{12} and B_6 may contribute to depression, anxiety, and memory issues. These symptoms often reverse after a patient starts the GFD and begins absorbing nutrients properly. (Note: It's easy to self-medicate when it comes to vitamins. You can buy them without a prescription. But please don't do that. Too much folate, B_6, or B_{12} can be dangerous. Be sure to consult your health-care provider.)

Several researchers have been talking about a connection between schizophrenia and gluten, too. While studies have shown that there is nothing to suggest that celiac disease and schizophrenia are linked, some research shows increased antibodies to gluten but not to celiac disease in patients with this mental disorder.[5] At least one recent study shows that gluten plays a possible role in some schizophrenia patients who had elevated TG6, the brain expression of gluten antibodies also being investigated as a marker for gluten ataxia (see page 46).[6] And some report an improvement in patients with schizophrenia once gluten is removed.

Such books as *Grain Brain* make a compelling argument for a relationship between gut inflammation caused by wheat and depression, anxiety, and Alzheimer's—even for people who don't have celiac disease.

Osteoporosis: It's Complicated

You might think that only older, postmenopausal women are candidates for osteoporosis and its precursor, osteopenia. But that's not true when it comes to celiac disease and dermatitis herpetiformis (for more on DH, see page 42). The small intestine is responsible for absorbing important nutrients, such as calcium, which is essential for building healthy bones. But it can't do its work when the intestine is damaged. Regardless of age or gender, someone with undiagnosed celiac disease or DH most likely will not get enough calcium to keep bones healthy even when taking calcium supplements. The calcium can't be absorbed properly.

Low bone density is common in children and adults who are untreated or newly diagnosed. In fact, bone loss was found in 58 percent of newly diagnosed children. In most cases and especially when the children were under the age of four, bone density returned to normal after they began a GFD.

One study found that 3 to 5 percent of osteoporosis patients had celiac disease compared to 0.5 percent in those with normal bone density. Men with celiac disease also need to be concerned about osteoporosis and bone health.

The good news is that for most celiac patients, when gluten is removed and the intestine begins to heal, normal absorption is restored and bone density will often improve.

People who are gluten sensitive will not be more susceptible to low blood calcium and low bone density than the general population.

To maintain bone health, the National Institutes of Health sets the following levels of vitamin D, calcium, and magnesium (for adults).

- Vitamin D (800 to 1,200 IUs)
- Calcium (1,000 mg for men and 1,200 mg for women)
- Magnesium (400 mg for men and 320 mg for women)

In addition, some patients, especially older adults, might need to take medication to help increase bone density.

Acid Redux

Let's face it. Heartburn and acid reflux are no strangers to folks with celiac disease.

But what's this topic doing in the middle of a discussion about bone density? The type of acid reflux medication you take may affect the absorption of calcium.

Once your blood calcium is at a normal level, meaning you are absorbing calcium properly, your physician might put you on a bisphosphonate class of medication (such as Actonel, Fosamax, or Boniva) to help stimulate bone growth or slow the loss of bone mass. But here are some things you need to know that might give you more heartburn.

These medications can cause acid reflux. And so your physician might recommend that you take one of the well-known acid reflux medications. Now you are on medication to build bone mass and taking calcium besides. And you are adding something to prevent acid reflux.

But here's a word of caution about some medications used to treat heartburn. In May 2011, the Food and Drug Administration (FDA) issued a statement warning consumers and health-care professionals that long-term or high-dose use of proton pump inhibitor (PPI) medications (such as Nexium, Prevacid, and Prilosec OTC) may increase the risk of bone fractures. That's because PPIs block the gastric acids, which play an important role in absorbing calcium in the small intestine. Therefore long-term use of these drugs has a detrimental effect on bone health, the FDA says.[7]

Histamine or H2 blockers (such as Zantac, Pepcid, and Tagamet) were not included in the FDA study because they reduce acid production by a different mechanism than is behind the PPIs.

What's a Person to Do?

Most physicians are not startled by this information (like I am) and suggest simply taking an additional calcium supplement to counter these effects. This is a situation where you and your doctor together will make the decision about what's best for your overall health and the health of your bones.

If you are on a PPI or considering them, ask your physician if one of the H2 medications might be a suitable substitute for you. And consider once-a-year bone density injections. These do not cause acid reflux, but they do have other risks. Yes, sometimes managing celiac disease is a revolving door.

Can Celiac Disease Cause Early Death?

Years of eating doughnuts and Danish pastries can do more than add on pounds. If you have celiac disease or one of the related autoimmune disorders, it stirs up all those T-cells, increasing the chances of having non-Hodgkin's lymphoma, other lymphomas, cancer of the small intestine, and other autoimmune diseases.

I know this sounds technical and worrisome. I don't mean to alarm you, but some recent studies found an increase in lymphomas and other cancers in people who went undiagnosed with celiac disease for many years or who did not stick to the gluten-free diet. One study, involving more than ten thousand Swedish patients who were hospitalized with celiac disease, found twice the rate of early death in these folks due to additional complications from celiac disease.

The study suggested that this may be due to reduced absorption of important nutrients, such as vitamins A and E. There is a silver lining to this study. It found that babies and toddlers hospitalized with celiac disease before age two had a reduced death risk. So, there might be benefits to being diagnosed and starting the gluten-free diet early in life.[8]

Another study of more than 7,600 celiac patients done in 2013, found people who still had signs of inflammation five years after they were diagnosed had 3.8 times the chance of being diagnosed with lymphoma.

Okay, take a deep breath. The numbers are still small, but anytime I hear the words *lymphoma* and *celiac disease* in the same sentence, it sends shivers through my DNA. The good news is that the risk goes down once gluten is removed from one's diet. I hope you are getting my drift here. *It is not healthy to cheat on your GFD.*

Reproductive Issues: Infertility, Pregnancy, and Miscarriage

Here's some info that may really surprise you—celiac disease can affect your fertility. Women with undiagnosed celiac disease have a two to four times' increased risk of infertility, spontaneous abortions, preterm deliveries, and delivery of low-birth-weight infants. Much of this may be because of severe vitamin deficiencies and anemia, the result of malabsorption that occurs in undiagnosed celiac disease. An Italian study on reproductive issues and women with celiac disease showed that some 65 percent of celiac patients reported at least one gestational disorder, compared to 31 percent of women without celiac disease.

There's good news, though: one of the conclusions of the study was that physicians should consider screening women with unexplained pregnancy problems and other reproductive issues, as the GFD might help prevent future complications.[9]

But what about men with undiagnosed celiac disease? Studies also suggest that men should also be screened for celiac disease when fertility issues cannot be otherwise explained.

Your Chance of Passing on the Genes

Many doctors still don't know that people with first-degree relatives who are celiac have a 1 in 22 chance of also having celiac disease. Your relatives (parent, child, sibling) should be tested, as well as second-degree relatives.

"I am shocked that more primary care doctors don't know this," says the NFCA's Alice Bast. But getting those first-degree relatives to the doctor can be tough, especially if they don't feel sick. Alice says when her initial requests didn't work, she explained some of the more frightening long-term risks, such as cancer, to get her family members tested.

Bob's Story:
A Doctor, a Celiac Patient, and a Celiac Parent

Bob is a board-certified gastroenterologist who was diagnosed with type 1 diabetes when he was a teenager. He recalls that he ate gluten-free bread as a child, but then he stopped and doesn't remember why.

He had been practicing medicine for many years when his daughter, who was seventeen at the time, developed night blindness. A complete medical workup was done but nothing definitive was ever found. Stephanie began losing weight during her first year at college and had become so thin, Bob hardly recognized her when he picked her up at the airport during one school break. She was very tired and very anemic.

After ruling out the bad stuff, a hematologist researched causes of unexplained anemia and celiac disease popped up. It turned out, she tested positive. This was in 2003, just about the time the prevalence study was being released.

Now it was Bob's turn to delve more deeply into the medical details of celiac disease, and he discovered both the genetic component and relationship to type 1 diabetes. He had himself tested and was also positive for celiac disease.

Today, he is an expert on celiac disease who sees a number of patients with celiac disease and gluten sensitivity. "Because I have celiac disease and type 1 diabetes, I think I have more empathy. I'm not apt to dismiss them as having anxiety or depression before I work them up and can rule out physical ailments like celiac disease."

He is particularly mindful of the genetic component of celiac disease and will run the blood tests on any patient who has a first-degree relative with celiac disease, Down syndrome, Turner syndrome, type 1 diabetes, elevated liver enzymes, anemia, or Hashimoto's disease.

He notes that, within the medical community, primary care physicians need more education. "I am seeing a lot of patients who are already on the diet when they come to me. They tell me their primary care doctor suggested they give it a try. Then I have to work backward to get a diagnosis or try to rule out celiac disease through genetic testing."

He sees two big challenges for his patients: (1) explaining the symptoms to a doctor when most adults don't really have the classic GI symptoms, and (2) sticking to the diet when they've been diagnosed.

"There are so many good gluten-free options now," says Bob, who always gives his patients a pep talk and tells them they can go out and enjoy themselves. "You can't isolate yourself because of this diet. That's not healthy, either. And it's not like I don't know. I live that way, too."

Today, Stephanie is very healthy and the mother of two young children, with twins on the way. So far, her children are free of celiac symptoms.

Symptoms of Celiac Disease in Babies and Children: Is there a Difference?

Less than twenty years ago, physicians thought celiac disease was a childhood condition characterized by low weight and short stature, distended belly, and diarrhea or large, foul-smelling stool. Today pediatricians look for a wide range of symptoms that include:

- Overweight
- Underweight
- Low stature
- Irritability
- Difficulty concentrating in school
- Diarrhea
- Constipation
- Pale complexion
- Abdominal pain
- Bloating
- Gas

Because symptoms in children are often subtle and mimic other intestinal diseases, such as irritable bowel syndrome (IBS) or lactose intolerance, the disease is often difficult to diagnose. Some children experience symptoms the first time they are exposed to gluten, whereas others develop symptoms later in life.

Babies and toddlers can only react and let you know there are battles raging inside them with such symptoms as overflowing, smelly diapers; inconsolable screaming; listlessness that seems to start a couple of hours after breakfast and gets worse as the day goes on; or exploding rage over small things so that a parent or physician might say, "This one has quite a temper."

Older children can verbalize what they are feeling. If your child continuously complains about tummy aches or headaches or feeling tired, and there is no apparent reason (cold, flu, or other virus), it's time to take notice.

Gut Reaction: A Family Story

My mother had high expectations for me, her firstborn daughter. A romantic at heart, she named me after Beth, a protagonist in *Little Women*, introduced me to classical music, and gave me piano lessons. She enrolled me in ballet and tap lessons at the local YMCA.

I wore a sparkly red, white, and blue sequined tutu for my first tap recital. I was five. I loved the costume. We stood in a row, all the little dancers, and practiced scuffing our tap shoes against the hard wood floor to produce that wonderful staccato sound, the mark of a true tap dancer.

But I hated dance lessons. As we stood in a line, shoulder to shoulder, the dance teacher always singled me out: "Beth, stand up straight. Suck in your belly."

Hard as I tried, I could do neither. My slender frame had the traditional weak muscles and protruding belly of a child with celiac disease. Although I was never heavy, my body image is forever cast as that of a five-year-old in a little red, white, and blue leotard, with a big, protruding belly.

Like many children, I was unable to vocalize my symptoms except to say, "My tummy hurts."

I self-medicated with food. When it was my turn to put away the leftovers after meals, most never made it from the table to the refrigerator. I was always hungry, eating frequently, trying to curb the disquiet inside me.

I should have remembered this part of my childhood when my son, Jeremy, was born. But as a child living with this disease, I had only

▶

▼

seen it from the inside out. As a parent, I was looking at it from the outside in.

What I saw was my son flopping from one piece of furniture to another. As the day wore on, the flopping got noticeably worse. His attention, very focused in the morning, unraveled later in the day, causing me to think he was reacting to something he was eating. He filled his diapers to overflowing with runny bowel movements. He butted people and things in an almost autistic-like manner and had a hard time relating to schoolmates. Because he could focus, spoke well, and learned quickly, autism spectrum disorder did not seem like a label that fit. Neither did attention deficit disorder, although, when he entered kindergarten, that was suggested.

As accustomed as I was to surveying my intake when I did not feel well, I had a difficult time doing so with my son. When he was born, his pediatrician told me his likelihood of having celiac disease was not very high. Today we know that 1 in 22 first-degree relatives are likely to have the disease. So I looked for other possibilities. I perused the ingredients in packages of Quacker Crackers, Cheerios, and Cheetos, trying to find other common offenders—was it corn or milk? Could it be sugar or food dyes? All of them were potential candidates.

Looking back, I am surprised I did not consider the obvious culprit. I never suspected gluten.

Like most people, I believed celiac disease was a failure to thrive issue, whereas my son was in the 99th percentile for weight and height.

Yet I sensed his behavior deteriorating throughout the day as he consumed more gluten and dairy. I read a book about elimination diets. The author, Dr. William G. Crook, was one of the early believers that food allergies and behavior were connected. A pediatrician, he saw a connection between antibiotics, ear infections, and food allergy. My son had none of those. Still, the book explained elimination diets and food diaries. I thought it couldn't hurt to try. The gluten-free diet was the one I knew best and I was well equipped and had the pantry to carry this out.

Over February vacation the year that Jeremy was in kindergarten, he ate what I ate—no gluten. When he returned to school, I sent a note titled, "Please don't feed the Jer-Bear," in which I asked his teachers

▶

▼

not to feed him any treats. I asked them to let me know if a special event was coming up and told them I would send in something appropriate. They agreed.

As a calmer, happier child began to emerge, I wondered whether I was on to something. At the end of two weeks, I put him back on a regular, wheat-filled diet. I knew the diagnosis would only be circumstantial unless I had him tested.

A week later, when I was at his school, his teacher took me aside. "You've taken him off that diet, haven't you?" she said. "I can see the difference." Now I had an independent confirmation that I was on the right track.

I contacted a pediatric gastroenterologist at nearby Connecticut Children's Hospital who had been recommended by two people in my support group and by my pediatrician. He ran two "screening" tests and the results were inconclusive. I asked him to run the more specific tests for celiac. He didn't recommend it. "He's growing normally and he's healthy," said the doctor.

"Perhaps he hasn't been eating enough gluten," I offered. "Maybe he is eating too many of my foods," I said. "If you could just write the tests up, I will wait until the summer and make sure I stuff him with gluten. Then I'll have him tested." He agreed.

I didn't wait, however. And when we did the blood tests, they were positive for celiac disease.

"Well, you give me no choice with the elevated tests and the fact that you have it," the doctor told me. "I have to scope him. But I have to tell you there is not a one in a million chance he has the disease," he said reviewing his growth charts with me once again.

"Humor me," I said.

After the endoscope, he came out to give us an update. "I owe you an apology," he said. "Your son's intestine was 'scalloped'; I could see the damage with my naked eye."

From then on, Children's Hospital changed its protocol on the celiac profile. In addition, it began working with the attention deficit/hyperactivity disorder (ADHD) clinic to screen their patients for celiac disease as well.

What If Your Child Has No Symptoms or Very Subtle Symptoms?

Like so many things about raising kids, this one is kind of a paradox. Be concerned, but not too worried.

Watch for symptoms in young children, especially if the child has first-degree relatives with celiac disease. Behavioral and learning issues can be symptoms as well and these will be more apparent as your child reaches school age and interacts with others outside the immediate family.

Like so many other issues, when your child's health is at stake, this is another where you need to follow your gut for the sake of his or hers, as this is a period in life where your child needs all the vitamins and nutrients he or she can get.

You'll be visiting the pediatrician quite often anyway—vaccinations, checkups, ear infections. Talk about your concerns and make sure the two of you monitor your child's progress together. You'll do that anyway. If you hear yourself bringing up concerns repeatedly, that might be an indication to test your child. Be persistent.

Things to Discuss with Your Child's Pediatrician

- If your child is an infant, determine when you should introduce gluten to him or her (see page 32).
- Review your child's growth chart at each visit. Slowed growth patterns could be evidence of celiac disease.
- If your child has a first-degree relative with celiac disease, remind his or her physician that children with a first-degree relative should be screened for celiac disease after age six and before puberty, even if the child has no symptoms of the disease.
- Ask whether you should do genetic testing. (You could rule out celiac disease at any age if your child does not have the DQ2 or DQ8 gene. If he or she doesn't have either gene, you can check this off your list of things to worry about. See page 34 for more about genetic testing.)

- Discuss tummy troubles, frequent bouts of diarrhea, unexplained vomiting, changes in appetite, and whether these warrant testing your child's antibody levels. If your child is lethargic or having trouble focusing in school, ask about testing antibodies and also running blood tests for vitamin levels. (A vitamin deficiency can be the first sign of celiac disease.)
- Take notes for several weeks prior to your child's next doctor's visit. Record foods eaten, changes in behavior, interactions with peers, and reports from teachers or day care providers.

Suddenly Celiac: Seniors and Celiac Disease

Nearly 30 percent of newly diagnosed celiac patients are over age sixty. So, if you think you or a parent or a great-aunt or uncle has dodged a bullet just because of being too old to have it, guess again.

There is no typical age for having celiac disease. You could have the genes, eat gluten all your life, and then suddenly start having symptoms. Life stresses, illness, a fall, or an accident are all thought of as possible triggers. Still other people might have vague symptoms for years before the diagnosis is made.

What's more, the symptoms in older patients are usually less digestive and more of the atypical symptoms, such as brain fog and fatigue, which can be easily attributed to aging.[10]

The Statistics

- According to the Mayo Clinic, the median age for diagnosing this disease is now age fifty.[11]
- Studies indicate that nearly 2 percent of older Americans have celiac disease; double the rate in the general population.
- One third of people in this group are diagnosed over the age of sixty.
- A small Israeli study found that the majority of symptoms were cognitive decline (Alzheimer's dementia-like symptoms) that improved on a gluten-free diet.[12]

The Good News and the Bad News

Seniors getting diagnosed say they feel ten to twenty years younger once they go gluten-free. And, hey, who doesn't want that? The bad news is, if someone has had undiagnosed celiac disease for many years, it will take longer for the gut to heal.

For seniors, adapting to a gluten-free diet can be challenging at best and overwhelming for some. Not only is the diet a major lifestyle adjustment, but it's one that might involve working with caregivers, retirement communities, and nursing homes, as well.

In addition, seniors tend to see more doctors and take more medications as they age, making this an additional challenge. All medications should be checked regularly and absorption (think: dosage) might change as the gut heals (see "Gluten and Medication," page 101).

Nevertheless, the improved quality of life is worth the effort. So stick with the diet, no matter what your age. And find an advocate to assist you in navigating the diet. A child, sibling, or perhaps a member of a local celiac support group can be an enormous help. Don't be afraid to ask.

What to Discuss with Your Physician

Traditional signs of aging that could actually be signs of celiac disease:

- I have intermittent brain fog. Sometimes I think I have dementia.
- I'm so tired all the time. I've had anemia all my life. My sister has celiac disease, but no one has ever tested me for it.
- I have osteoporosis. Is that a symptom of celiac disease?
- My husband passed away suddenly. I thought I was reacting to the shock of losing him, but it's been nearly a year and I still feel tired and draggy every day. I'd like to rule out other causes (such as celiac disease) for feeling so poorly.

Raising Your GF IQ:
Myths About Seniors and Celiac Disease

I'm too old to have this.

That's not true. Nearly 30 percent of newly diagnosed celiac patients are over the age of sixty. The incidence is about double the rate of the general population.

I've probably had this forever. It won't make any difference if I go on the diet now. So, why bother?

Aside from the newly found energy and feeling of well-being that most patients experience, symptoms of brain fog and confusion, often dismissed as dementia, will often improve once a celiac senior is following a gluten-free diet.

Other symptoms, such as osteoporosis and anemia, improved in patients followed in the Israeli study. This means the potential for increased energy and the potential for a lower risk of broken bones.

I can't expect the kitchen at a retirement facility to take care of my diet.

You can, and you should. As more of us reach that golden age and more people are diagnosed with celiac disease, institutional kitchens are learning to accommodate the gluten-free diet. Clear labeling and more choices of products make this a much easier request.

If you are shopping for a retirement facility, your checklist should include looking for a kitchen staff that is trained and can safely serve gluten-free food. A meeting with the director of food service should be part of the tour and you should discuss a protocol for who will serve you and how they will confirm that each meal has been prepared for your diet. *To be sure you are covered, make sure the contract has a clause that gluten-free meals will be provided.*

In fact, it's already happening. As this book went to press, four retirement communities in Washington State and two in Arizona had received Gluten-free Food Service accreditation, a program of the Gluten Intolerance Group of North America (GIG). GIG works with institutional kitchens throughout the United States to help them establish protocols for safely serving gluten-free guests. Look for this list to multiply as more baby boomers and more celiac patients enter the golden years.

Tips: If you are living in a retirement community or nursing home and diagnosed with celiac disease . . .

- Set up a meeting with the director of the facility, the head of food service, the staff social worker, and nurse, if the facility has them.
- Bring along an adult child, sibling, or your spouse.
- Discuss the diet and why it is so important to your health.
- Provide guidelines for the diet and review gluten-free options (see "National Support Group Organizations" on page 301).

2

Getting Tested for Celiac Disease

Nothing about celiac disease, or digestive issues, for that matter, is simple. Just as the symptoms mimic so many other ailments, the diagnostic process is complicated, too. Fortunately, testing is much easier and more reliable than it was when I was diagnosed. It starts with a blood test or a panel of blood tests.

If the tests are positive, the doctor recommends an endoscopy, the "gold standard" for diagnosing celiac disease, and takes a series of small tissue biopsies while you are comfortably sedated.

All of these tests and procedures are listed in the American College of Gastroenterology (ACG) guidelines for the diagnosis and management of celiac disease, available at the ACG website, gi.org.

Keep in mind these guidelines are not binding on physicians or insurance companies. Some of these tests are quite costly, and cheaper, effective blood tests may exist, so you'll need to talk with your doctor about the options and check with your health insurance company to verify what will be covered. Find out exactly what you will need to pay out-of-pocket as copayments or under your high deductible (HSA or Health Insurance Exchange) policy limits. Refer to the ACG guidelines if you run into problems with your insurer. Quest Diagnostics (questdiagnostics.com), a clinical lab service, has comprehensive guidelines and tests listed on its website.

The Blood Tests

The initial blood screening can be done by any physician who suspects you might have celiac disease. Your primary care physician is often the best place to start.

The screening blood tests measure the blood levels of antibodies, proteins normally produced by the immune system to fight off infection. The body can also produce antibodies to fight off foreign substances, such as allergens. If you have celiac disease, the body forms antibodies when you eat gluten. The specific blood tests your doctor will order will tell him or her whether your antibodies to gluten are elevated.

Don't worry about memorizing the names of these tests. It's just a good idea to read them once so you'll have some understanding about this complicated diagnosis.

Normally, your physician will run a blood test called TTG-IgA, the preferred single blood test for patients over age two. To break this down: TTG stands for tissue transglutaminase, an enzyme produced in the intestine. IgA, or immunoglobulin A, is an antibody our body produces to fight infection. If this test is positive, it indicates the body is creating antibodies to its own tissues, most likely in response to eating gluten. However, some people with celiac disease (5 to 10 percent) don't produce the normal amount of IgA, a condition called IgA deficiency. If you are IgA deficient, the TTG-IgA test may not be positive even if you have the condition. If the doctor suspects IgA deficiency, he or she may order the total IgA blood test at the same time. This test is used to determine IgA deficiency. The TTG-IgG test (IgG stands for immunoglobulin G, another antibody) and the DGP-IgG (deamidated gliadin peptides-immunoglobulin G) may be added at the same time. These are the best tests if someone has IgA deficiency.

For screening children under two years of age, TTG-IgA and DGP (IgA and IgG) should be ordered, as young children may not have had a chance to produce their own antibodies.

And there's one more thing. You must be eating gluten to get an accurate diagnosis. If you give up gluten first or reduce the amount you eat, your test results may be falsely negative because the body will have no reason to produce antibodies.

Typically the DGP blood test is more sensitive than TTG, and would become elevated sooner and return to normal more quickly. But one incidence of eating gluten will not cause any antibodies to become elevated. It's thought that the antibodies won't react unless a person eats gluten for two to four weeks, the time it takes for a new round of intestinal damage to occur.

Scientists at Stanford University Medical Center and elsewhere are looking at ways to shorten that period when a person needs to eat gluten in order to be tested. A team has now laid the groundwork for a way to diagnose celiac disease in a much shorter time—six days—and with a much-reduced gluten intake.[1]

Can I Have Celiac Disease If All the Tests Are Negative?

If the blood tests are all negative, it's possible you have an IgA deficiency, if the tests that your doctor ran were based on the IgA antibodies. If, however, you had a biopsy and it showed no villous atrophy (flattening or blunting of the villi), then it's pretty certain you don't have this disease.

If you still feel badly after eating gluten, you might have nonceliac gluten sensitivity or it's possible you could have a wheat allergy. Wheat allergy affects a very small percentage of people, but one of those people could be you.

Small Bowel Biopsy

If one or more of the blood tests show your antibodies are elevated, your physician will refer you to a gastroenterologist for definitive diagnosis. The gastroenterologist will perform a small bowel biopsy through endoscopy. The procedure is done under moderate sedation and takes about 20 minutes. Someone can drive you home shortly after you wake up. You may experience some discomfort the first day—bloating and a tiny bit of bleeding are not uncommon and not worrisome.

Celiac disease can cause patchy lesions in the duodenum (the upper-most portion of the small intestine), which can be missed if only one or two samples are taken, so it's best to take three or four biopsies to increase the detection to 95 percent and 100 percent, respectively. Some physicians will take as many as six biopsies. Verify that your physician will be taking several biopsies from different parts of your intestinal lining.

When Is the Right Time to Test Infants and Young Children?

Generally, physicians do not recommend screening infants and young children for celiac disease unless they are symptomatic. If a first-degree relative has celiac disease, then most of the leading physicians specializing in celiac disease recommend that children over the age of six be screened even if they have no symptoms and definitely before the onset of puberty.

Reliable Tests

Before the age of two, most children will not have fully developed their own antibodies to gluten. And testing can result in a false negative. That said, failure to thrive, explosive diarrhea, chronic colic or indigestion, and irritability are all signals that your child needs to be tested for celiac disease regardless of his age.

The recommended tests are TTG-IgA and DGP (IgA and IgG);[2] an elevated test should be confirmed with a small bowel biopsy (for more detail on these tests, see pages 30–32).

Introducing Gluten to a Baby

Should gluten be introduced after infancy, before weaning, sooner, later? Ah, this is another paradox about raising children. Pediatricians have been all over the place on this one. New findings indicate that breastfeeding while introducing gluten helps protect infants from celiac disease and perhaps even other autoimmune diseases and food sensitivities.

One of the leading theories is that breastfeeding promotes the growth of friendly bacteria in an infant's gut and that might prevent or delay the onset of celiac disease. Check out the article in the *New York Times* (February 2013) by Moises Velasquez-Manoff, titled "Who Has the Guts for Gluten?" It talks about an epidemic of celiac disease that struck Sweden between 1984 and 1996 when the Swedish government changed the guidelines on when to introduce gluten to infants. The government suggested waiting to introduce gluten until a baby was six months old, which was about the time most babies were being weaned. At the same time, companies had increased the amount of gluten in baby food. The result: the prevalence of celiac disease tripled to 3 percent.

Sweden then reversed its infant-feeding guidelines: keep breastfeeding, the government urged, while simultaneously introducing small amounts of gluten. The result, the epidemic abated.

Another study in the journal *Pediatrics* found a significantly reduced prevalence of celiac disease in a group of twelve-year-olds born in 1997, a year when experts recommended introducing gluten-containing products when babies were four months old and during a time when it was more common to breastfeed for a longer period of time. This prompted researchers to recommend introducing gluten slowly, beginning at four months of age (not six months) and to continue breastfeeding.[3]

Still it's not clear whether any of these recommendations (introducing gluten earlier rather than later, while breastfeeding, or after weaning) prevents celiac disease or simply delays the onset. In addition, not all subsequent studies have found nursing protective, but partly as a result of Sweden's experience, the American Academy of Pediatrics now recommends that infants start consuming gluten between four and six months and while still breastfeeding.[4]

It's also not clear that every pediatrician is aware of or follows this guideline. You'll need to discuss this with your child's physician.

"In a few months we will know the results of a gigantic prospective study conducted in Europe (called PreventCD) that will almost surely be a milestone in our understanding on what are the best infant feeding practices to help reduce the risk of celiac in genetically predisposed babies," says Dr. Stefano Guandalini, professor and section chief, Pediatric Gastroenterology, University of Chicago, and founder and medical director, Celiac Disease Center. In Resources, page 301, I list studies and articles that are relevant to this subject. You can find copies on the Internet. Print them out and take them to your child's pediatrician.

Genetic Tests and Why You May Want Them

Two genes have been identified in celiac disease, HLA-DQ2 and HLA-DQ8, sometimes stated only as DQ2 and DQ8. One or both need to be present to have celiac disease, but having these is not an indication that you will have the disease. In fact, according to the University of Chicago Celiac Disease Center website, one third of the population has the genes for celiac disease; however, only 1 to 4 percent of us will actually develop the disease.

Therefore, genetic testing is not a method for diagnosing celiac disease. But it can be used to rule it out. So, when is testing useful?

We talked about screening first-degree relatives. But people who test negative for the gene would not be required to have regular antibody screening. The chance of getting celiac disease without having one or both of the genes is slim to none. For example, the children of an adult with celiac disease could have the gene test. The results would allow the parent to know which children need close monitoring.

Testing is helpful for people who are already on the gluten-free diet, whereby antibody blood tests will always be negative. If someone tests negative for the celiac genes, he or she might still have gluten sensitivity, but eating gluten will not trigger an autoimmune response.

Because 35 percent of the American population have either DQ2 (more common) or DQ8, it is possible for two affected people to marry each other. The genes can be passed on by males as well as females, although the incidence of celiac disease is slightly higher in women. Therefore, one person's gene test doesn't necessarily mean that the other side of the family is not affected as well. And new research is examining these gene pairs and how various combinations might affect a patient's symptoms.

For more information about genetic tests for celiac disease visit the University of Chicago Celiac Disease Center website (cureceliac.org) and search for "genetic testing."

Note that, unlike the antibody testing for which you must be eating gluten to get an accurate result, it's not necessary for genetic testing. The genes are part of your DNA.

Raising Your GF IQ:
Some Common Questions About Genetic Testing

If my child has both genes for celiac disease, but I only have one of them, does that mean the other gene came from the other parent?

The genes for celiac disease are not dominant and recessive. A person can have DQ2, DQ8, or both, and still be at risk for the disease. Genes are either passed from parents to child or not. If a child has both genes and a particular parent only has one, then the other gene must have been passed from the other parent.

If both parents test negative for the celiac genes, does that mean their children are also negative?

Yes, the children of two persons who don't have the genes for celiac disease will also be free of the genes for the disease.

Follow-up:
If Celiac Disease Is Positive, Now What?

If your small bowel biopsy is positive, your doctor will recommend a strict gluten-free diet because it's currently the only treatment for celiac disease. You won't receive any medications, no pills, no shots. But you will need to be hypervigilant about what you put in your mouth. It's all in your hands, my friend. The next two parts of this book will help you navigate staying on this diet and living well.

Your physician will need to check out your overall health, including blood calcium levels, bone density, and thyroid levels. He or she should also run vitamin and mineral panels, as many newly diagnosed patients have low levels of vitamins B_{12}, B_6, and D, and iron, folic acid, copper, zinc, and carnitine.

Once you begin the diet, your primary care physician or gastroenterologist can monitor your overall health. About six months after you are diagnosed, the doctor will probably repeat the blood test. If you have been following a gluten-free diet, the results should be closer to normal. He or she will continue to run this blood test (every few months) until the numbers are in the normal range; then repeat them each year or two to make sure you are sticking to the diet.

After your gut begins to heal, you will likely notice some weight gain that might not make you happy, but your doctor will be delighted. That signals that the villi are growing back (they will do that) and you are absorbing food properly. So, if you feel like celebrating the new gluten-free you, don't do it with a new wardrobe until you've settled into a healthy routine of good, gluten-free food and exercise.

Your medications might also be better absorbed, which means your doctor will need to adjust the dosage of some of the medicines you take. Thyroid medication, insulin, blood thinners, cholesterol medications, and antidepressants are among the likely candidates that will need to be reviewed.

If you have persistent symptoms despite the diet, you might go back to the gastroenterologist for more follow-up tests, but you don't need another endoscopy unless you continue having problems. Some patients and their doctors prefer to have an annual follow-up with the gastroenterologist; other patients feel comfortable being followed by their primary care physician. It's a personal choice and one that might also depend on your insurance benefits and your comfort level with each doctor.

Once the antibody levels are negative, you should have an annual blood test to make sure the antibodies continue to stay in the normal range, an indication you are not cheating on the gluten-free diet. Only one blood test is necessary (usually the DGP or TTG). Make this part of your annual checklist and checkup. It's a good way to make sure that you are not accidentally getting gluten-ed. And make sure your doctor continues to check your vitamin levels, too. If you are low in iron, B vitamins, calcium, or vitamin D, your doctor may suggest supplements (see page 101) and may want to check your antibody levels again to make sure you are sticking to the diet. This doesn't mean you are secretly eating pizza. Sometimes gluten can sneak into your diet through medication or cross-contamination, too.

Use the follow-up blood test as a way to monitor your child's compliance with the diet, too. It's especially useful when you suspect a rebellious teenager is straying. Parents can be wrong, but science can't be ignored.

Timing: Testing, Diagnosis, and Healing

Not even a decade ago, if you had celiac symptoms, you could go for up to eleven years before a doctor figured out what ailed you. According to Peter H. R. Green, MD, director, Celiac Disease Center, Columbia University College of Physicians and Surgeons, it still takes an average of four years from onset of symptoms to diagnosis in the United States. That's a big improvement.

And yet, as Dr. Green says, "There's still room for improvement in this area. There certainly needs to be more work done in educating physicians about how common the disease is and how it is diagnosed."

The length of time to full recovery depends on your age at diagnosis and length of time between symptoms and diagnosis. Upon starting a gluten-free diet, most people notice some relief almost immediately and the gut begins to heal within a couple of weeks. (It also depends on how carefully you stick to the diet.)

When You Don't Get Better: Refractory Sprue

When you are doing everything right and you still have ongoing diarrhea and your most recent biopsy still shows villous atrophy (flattened villi), you may have refractory sprue. I don't want to scare you, but this is a very serious condition that can lead to cancer. Primary refractory sprue is when symptoms persist despite following the GFD. As Dr. Green notes in *Celiac Disease: A Hidden Epidemic*, this is a diagnosis of exclusion when other conditions, such as pancreatic insufficiency, bacterial overgrowth, microscopic colitis, and small intestinal lymphoma, have been ruled out.

There's also a condition called secondary refractory sprue, which occurs when a person is initially doing well on the GFD, then has a relapse despite following the diet. In this case, other treatments may be used, including steroids, immunosuppressive therapy, and antibiotics. Sometimes the person may be hospitalized and treated with intravenous fluids and nutrients, says Dr. Green.[5]

Both conditions occur very infrequently, but it's good to know about them in case you have persistent symptoms after you've been diagnosed.

While treatments for this condition are limited, the future is looking brighter for folks with this debilitating condition. Research and clinical trials for a new drug are taking place under Dr. Thomas Waldmann at the National Institutes of Health and Dr. Joseph Murray at the Mayo Clinic. The experimental drug aims at reversing tissue damage from gluten and can potentially accelerate healing in patients with refractory sprue.

Raising Your GF IQ: Frequently Asked Questions About Testing and Diagnosis

What is the difference between latent and silent celiac disease?

Silent celiac disease is when you have no symptoms but test positive for antibodies and a small intestine biopsy is positive. Many people with celiac disease have no outward symptoms. Often the doctor tests you because of secondary issues, such as osteoporosis, infertility, and unexplained anemia, which are not improving.

Latent celiac disease is when a person tests positive for one celiac antibody but has no intestinal damage when a biopsy is done. If you are told you have latent celiac disease, this means you are at risk for developing the disease and should be monitored regularly by your doctor.

I had silent symptoms before being diagnosed with celiac disease. Now I have a two-year-old son. He has no celiac symptoms. Should I have him tested and, if so, when?

Blood testing for celiac antibodies (TTG-IgA) might be falsely negative below age two. So, children at risk for celiac disease but without symptoms usually are not tested until after their second birthday. Because he is the first-degree relative of someone with celiac disease, he should be tested in the next few years and before the onset of puberty. If the tests are negative, he should still be watched closely, as celiac disease can present at any age. Alternatively, if genetic testing indicates he does not have the genes for celiac disease, you won't need to worry about monitoring him for this condition.

Can a stool test tell me whether I have celiac disease or gluten sensitivity?

Leading celiac medical experts believe the stool test is not a reliable method for diagnosing celiac disease or gluten sensitivity despite claims by these labs to the contrary. To date, the findings on using this method of testing have not been peer reviewed and are not recommended by mainstream medical doctors. Nevertheless, a number of patients who believe they're reacting to gluten turn to a stool test as a method of gluten sensitivity testing and report feeling much better once they eliminate gluten.

Can my doctor test me for celiac disease when I have a colonoscopy?

Ouch! I'm afraid I've heard this one more than once. Celiac disease takes place in the duodenum or top portion of the small intestine. You'd need a very long, very flexible tube and high tolerance for pain to have the procedure done through colonoscopy. And if your doctor thinks he can find celiac disease in the colon, think again. Celiac disease is also called villous atrophy because the villi are blunted or flattened. There are *no* villi in the large intestine.

Note: You still need to have routine screening colonoscopy performed to rule out colon cancer, just like all other adults.

What about home tests? Can I test myself for celiac disease?

Home testing of products and people (gene and serology) are readily available. Maybe your motivation is to save some money by avoiding going to a doctor or because you don't have health insurance or it does not cover testing. The issue is in the quality of the testing and interpretation. You can get into trouble by acting on false negatives or positives. So, while these tests may prove useful, just know their limitations.

3

A Broader Spectrum of Gluten-Related Disorders

Isn't it amazing that something you eat could affect your brain, eyes, skin, or mental acuity? Such is the complex story of gluten. Personally I have always thought of gluten and gut in the same breath because my symptoms when I am gluten-ed are bellyaches and heartburn. The cause and effect helps me monitor my own diet and stay clear of gluten.

But gluten can cause some very strange and not-so-obvious symptoms in other parts of the body without causing digestive symptoms. However, absorption in those intestinal walls is how it all starts. You could say, the small intestine is the sun in our solar system.

Why and how this takes place is the focus of this section. Although celiac disease was the first gluten-related condition to be identified, it's certainly not the last. Leading research doctors in this field have identified a whole spectrum of gluten-related disorders and they wrote about them in a paper released in 2012.

In it, they question why this dietary protein (gluten) is so toxic to so many people and talk about the wide range of adverse reactions being reported. The authors speculate that it's due to the production over the last ten thousand years of wheat varieties with higher gluten content, and they theorize that some people are more vulnerable to this protein, having never adequately adapted to gluten.

In addition to celiac disease, the spectrum of disorders in the paper includes dermatitis herpetiformis (DH), gluten ataxia, gluten sensitivity, and wheat allergy.[1]

We'll talk about those momentarily, but first, I'd be remiss if I didn't mention the 800-pound gluten-free gorilla that has millions avoiding gluten these days. Outside of the medical papers on the topic of gluten and how it affects every part of the body, health professionals, food chemists, and best-selling authors are linking gluten to everything from high blood sugar to heart disease, Alzheimer's disease, and dementia. One theory points to genetically modified organisms (GMOs); some scientists believe these are why wheat (soy and corn, too) triggers the reactions responsible for ailments although most experts agree that wheat is not genetically modified in this country. Others speculate that the hybridization of wheat is to blame. Or perhaps it's a more pesticide resistant wheat crop, higher gluten content in today's wheat or that people were never meant to digest it to begin with. These are all leading theories.

And other parts of the wheat are being looked at as culprits, too. You'll hear these buzzwords: *lectins* (specific carbohydrate-binding proteins), *fructans* (short-chain fructose/sugar molecules), and something called *amylase trypsin inhibitors* (ATIs), a protein in wheat that naturally protects the plant against pests. It's a lot to digest.

While scientific research is limited, speculation grows everyday that these are causes for many wheat-related concerns. These are becoming hot buttons in the gluten-free world.

And you'll notice some overlap in the symptoms and conditions in this chapter as we delve into what you need to know about the spectrum of gluten-related conditions as identified by leading medical researchers.

Dermatitis Herpetiformis

Dermatitis herpetiformis (DH) is an itchy, blistering rash, often on the elbows and knees, which is associated with celiac disease. It is a skin form of CD. Usually the rash is symmetrical, appearing on both sides of the body.

It is not known why only some patients with celiac disease develop DH and what factors link the two.

Only a small number of patients (about 10 percent) have gastrointestinal symptoms, and these are usually mild. However, more than half of DH patients also have celiac-type villous atrophy.[2] DH patients may have the same associated disorders as patients with celiac disease, such as autoimmune diseases, iron-deficient anemia, osteoporosis, and cancer.[3]

A skin biopsy is considered the "gold standard" for diagnosing DH. This is performed on uninvolved skin adjacent to the affected area. As DH is the skin version of celiac disease, a positive skin biopsy means the patient often does not need an intestinal biopsy. In fact, blood tests and an intestinal biopsy may not always accurately diagnose celiac disease in DH patients. Nevertheless, a strict gluten-free diet is the treatment.

Even though this is a form of celiac disease and triggered by gluten, it's all about the skin. A dermatologist is your best bet when it comes to diagnosing this condition. He or she can test you by taking a biopsy of the skin and testing for TTG-IgA antibodies. Some physicians will also recommend performing an intestinal biopsy to assess intestinal damage.

Raising Your GF IQ:
Things to Know About Living with DH

- Certain drugs and foods exacerbate DH and should be avoided. These may include NSAIDs (anti-inflammatory medications) and iodine. For some reason, people with DH lesions often have a sensitivity to iodine and the skin will not heal until iodine is minimized. This includes avoiding iodized salt, seafood, and seaweed.
- People with DH must follow a gluten-free diet for their well-being.
- Blisters and itching are often treated with Dapsone, or topical creams (cortisone).
- Once the skin has healed, it is not necessary to avoid skin creams that contain gluten.

Follow-up

Just as the diagnosis can be more complicated, the guidelines for follow-up testing for patients with DH are less specific than they are for celiac disease. So I asked one of the leading experts, gastro-enterologist Joseph A. Murray, MD (Mayo Clinic Department of Gastroenterology and Hepatology, Rochester, Minnesota). Here's what he suggests.

- If you require Dapsone, then regular blood tests for side effects of Dapsone are needed.
- At least once a year, repeat the TTG-IgA. Once you get off Dapsone, monitor for rash recurrence and repeat the TTG-IgA once a year or every other year as follow-up once the test is negative.
- If the first gut biopsy shows damage to the villi, then an intestinal biopsy should be repeated in two years after beginning the GFD.
- No follow-up biopsy is necessary if the first one is negative.

Bottom line

Start with the physician who diagnosed you. Most likely, that will be a dermatologist or a gastroenterologist. Discuss the best ways to monitor your health. Bring this page with you as a checklist to begin that dialogue and to help map out a plan of action.

A GFD Is Important for Anyone with DH

Unlike celiac disease, the itchy blisters associated with DH can be treated with medication that gives you some relief. Once they are managed, you might start thinking, "My symptoms are virtually gone, so why bother with the gluten-free diet?"

Don't fall for that line of thinking. DH is an autoimmune disease triggered by gluten. Eating it causes an autoimmune response, just like celiac disease. A gluten-free diet is really the treatment for DH; Dapsone and topical creams are meant only to minimize the symptoms. Besides,

Dapsone is a strong medication that can have side effects. So stick to your GFD.

Gluten on the Brain:
Neurological Conditions Caused by Gluten

Lately, medical experts are linking gluten to all kinds of brain and neurological issues from tingling sensations in the fingers and toes (neuropathy) to balance issues, wandering or "swimming" eyes, difficulty focusing, brain fog, and forgetfulness.

So if you are feeling clumsy, bumping into walls, forgetful, suffering brain fog, or experiencing tingling in your fingers or toes, you'll want to read this section.

Peripheral Neuropathy

About 10 percent of newly diagnosed celiac patients have a neurological condition and most often it is peripheral neuropathy. You know that sensation that your foot has fallen asleep or the tingling, pins-and-needles sensations you might get? Those are what people with peripheral neuropathy have. Besides celiac disease, it is also reported in people with gluten sensitivity.

Peripheral neuropathy, caused by nerve damage, actually is one of the most common nondigestive symptoms of celiac disease, according to the University of Chicago Celiac Disease Center. In fact, peripheral neuropathy and other neurological symptoms (balance, brain fog) may be the reason some people are diagnosed with celiac disease.

The good news is that symptoms of peripheral neuropathy can resolve or improve once the patient removes gluten from his or her diet.

Epilepsy

About 3 to 5 percent of celiac patients, mostly children and older adults, also have epilepsy. It's unclear whether the two conditions are related, but anecdotal reports say the frequency and degree of seizures may improve when these patients begin a GFD.

Migraines

Those blazing headaches that make you feel like your head is in a vice can be a symptom of celiac disease. According to one study, 4 percent of migraine patients had celiac disease. Other, less severe headaches are also common and a frequent symptom in patients with gluten sensitivity. Both groups say their headaches improve or disappear once they begin a GFD.

Gluten Ataxia

Gluten ataxia is an autoimmune neurological condition involving the body's reaction to gluten. Instead of in the gut, the response takes place in the brain, specifically the cerebellum, and can cause problems with gait, gross motor skills coordination, judging distance, tremor, and eye movement.

Sometimes the damage can be permanent. Once a diagnosis is made, patients are advised to stay on a very strict gluten-free diet for life. However, because gluten ataxia is relatively new, and not all physicians agree that it exists, there's very little research on this condition. In addition, it affects only a small segment of people and most often the symptoms are subtle.

Marios Hadjivassiliou, MD, a neurologist at Royal Hallamshire Hospital in Sheffield, England, first described gluten ataxia in the 1990s when he started testing for gluten sensitivity in patients who came to him with unexplained balance and coordination issues. Dr. Hadjivassiliou made some interesting observations, too. He wrote that celiac disease, DH, and gluten ataxia are all manifestations of gluten sensitivity but are different diseases. He also reported that gluten sensitivity is not principally a disease of the small bowel and that it can be primarily and sometimes only a neurological disease.

Diagnosis and Follow-up

Today, gluten ataxia is often a diagnosis of exclusion, diagnosed (by a neurologist) when antigliadin tests suggest gluten sensitivity and when other causes of ataxia are ruled out. A small bowel biopsy is recommended for patients with positive antigliadin and celiac blood tests. Dr. Hadjivassiliou also noticed that patients with gluten ataxia had an antibody, serum anti-transglutaminase-6 (TG6), the specific antibody to gluten that shows up in the brain. The test for TG6 is just starting to be used in the United States as a tool for diagnosing gluten ataxia.

Because prolonged exposure to gluten can cause irreversible damage in patients with gluten ataxia, a GFD is started immediately after diagnosis and patients should be followed closely by their physician. Blood tests should be repeated often (the timing depends on each patient) to make sure the antibodies are negative. In addition to diet, physical and occupational therapy may be prescribed.

Okay, if you are like me, you probably think you have this because you've been bumping into the same counter for three days or dropping your cell phone every time you pick it up. Relax. Ataxia in all forms is a fairly rare condition, affecting only 8.4 people out of every 100,000 in the United States. This means fewer still actually have gluten ataxia, about 2,990 to 10,660 people total in the United States.

Still, if you have concerns, discuss this with your doctor. Early intervention is key with gluten ataxia and it's very important to follow a strict gluten-free diet at all times.

Gluten Sensitivity

> Personally, I think gluten sensitivity is what we called chronic fatigue twenty years ago.
>
> —Robert G. Schwartz, MD, gastroenterologist

Are you reading this and thinking, "I know gluten is making me sick," even though your tests for celiac disease keep coming back negative. Maybe you are one of the growing number of folks who have gluten sensitivity. It's one more area in which gluten may be responsible for any number of ailments, although the connection is just starting to be acknowledged among medical folks.

It is now becoming evident that, besides celiac disease and wheat allergy (see page 52), there are people who react to gluten and for whom neither allergic nor autoimmune mechanisms can be identified. This is now called nonceliac gluten sensitivity or gluten sensitivity.

Gluten sensitivity is a relatively new medical condition. It is considered a condition of exclusion, usually diagnosed by eliminating the possibility of a wheat allergy or celiac disease. Simply put, you experience distress when eating gluten and show improvement when following a GFD. A gluten challenge (reintroducing gluten into your diet) is most often used to evaluate whether your health improves with the elimination or reduction of gluten. Currently there are no tests that are specific for gluten sensitivity. But research is under way.

The symptoms for gluten sensitivity may resemble those associated with celiac disease: abdominal pain; eczema and/or rash; headache; clumsiness; foggy mind; fatigue; diarrhea; depression; anemia; numbness in the legs, arms, or fingers; and joint pain. Interestingly, classic symptoms include diarrhea, bloating, or constipation, but no obvious intestinal damage seems to show up when patients are tested for celiac disease.

The Prevalence

It's possible that the number of people with gluten sensitivity is much higher than that of celiac disease. At first, some medical researchers speculated that the numbers of gluten-sensitive patients was between 18 to 20 million. But without medical tests to definitively diagnose gluten sensitivity, these numbers cannot be supported. Medical researchers are looking at developing tools to better diagnose and project the size of the gluten sensitive population.

Meanwhile some medical researchers believe that between 3 and 6 percent of the population may have nonceliac gluten sensitivity; others suspect the number is closer to 1 percent.

Gluten sensitivity was a hot button at the International Celiac Disease Symposium hosted by the University of Chicago in September 2013. In the next few years, this condition will most likely move to the center of the plate, right next to celiac disease.

What Gluten Sensitivity Is Not

While celiac disease and nonceliac gluten sensitivity share some common symptoms, gluten sensitivity is a condition distinct from celiac disease.

Gluten sensitivity does not cause an autoimmune reaction to gluten, or damage to the small intestine. Gluten sensitivity is also not associated with HLA genes as is celiac disease. Patients do not test positive for allergic response to wheat (see "Wheat Allergy," page 52). Essentially it's diagnosed by ruling out these other conditions.

Who Can Diagnose Me?

Few doctors are familiar with gluten sensitivity. And without a specific test for this condition, the subset of physicians who might tackle your issues is small. Find someone who you can speak to comfortably and who is receptive to research you may provide, as this may become a team effort. You may want to consult your primary care physician and a gastroenterologist first to help you rule out celiac disease, and you might go to an allergist to rule out wheat allergy.

What if you excluded celiac disease and wheat allergy, but you are still having the annoying symptoms that sent you to the doctor in the first place? Your best medical ally might be a naturopathic physician. Many specialize in gluten-related issues and the gluten-free diet. While I don't advocate "alternative" medicine as the primary method of diagnosis, it might provide you with a solution if traditional medicine has not. For a list of nationally known naturopathic physicians, see Resources, page 307. Many insurance carriers will not cover nontraditional treatments for gluten sensitivity. Check first to avoid surprise expenses.

Or like many people, you might decide to adopt a gluten-free diet on your own. The relief from symptoms might be enough to confirm that you have gluten sensitivity.

Gluten Sensitivity, Seniors, and Kids

Seniors

As you can imagine, there's very little data on this new condition—even less as it pertains to seniors and kids. But we do know that gluten sensitivity seems to be more prevalent in adults than in children. And it's possible that senior adults for whom celiac disease has been ruled out, might suffer from gluten sensitivity and benefit from the gluten-free diet.

But here's the rub. Physicians who treat elderly patients don't usually recommend the GFD unless there is a specific medical diagnosis. This could be changing as more research is done on gluten sensitivity. But until then, this is another situation where you'll want to arm yourself with medical studies and discuss this with your doctor.

Kids

Because evidence of a gluten sensitivity is largely anecdotal, kids won't have the years of symptoms and stories that would lead a parent or doctor to diagnose gluten sensitivity, so there are just not a lot of data on this, either.

According to Dr. Guandalini, the current thinking is that it is more common in adults, but the prevalence is really not known. "I myself have perhaps a handful—no more—of children who seem to fulfill this definition. Some have GI issues (abdominal bloating, discomfort, constipation on/off), others have headaches, one has major behavioral issues. But then again, the diagnosis only rests on patient's history, and in the case of children, only on parents' report of such history," he reports.

Irritable Bowel Syndrome (IBS): Another Masquerader

As if sorting out your digestive issues is not complicated enough, IBS, a functional disorder of the gastrointestinal tract, mimics many of the symptoms in gluten sensitivity, colitis, Crohn's disease, and celiac disease. It's been reported that a full 30 percent of folks with celiac disease are first diagnosed with IBS. IBS is often the first diagnosis of people with gluten sensitivity as well. To make this more confusing, IBS can exist along with these other conditions, as symptoms include bloating, diarrhea and/or constipation, tummy rumbles, and fatigue. Sound familiar? Often people have visited a number of doctors and had several endoscopies, colonoscopies, X-rays, blood tests, and such, but all testing is normal. It's another diagnosis of exclusion.

Traditionally, IBS is treated with diet modifications, probiotics and laxatives, antidiarrheals, antispasmodics, or bulking agents, but often these don't satisfactorily resolve the symptoms.

Now dietitians and physicians in the United States are looking at the low-FODMAP diet as an IBS treatment. And there is some initial evidence that FODMAP rather than gluten might be the culprit in many cases of gluten sensitivity.

FODMAP and Gluten Sensitivity: A Vowel Movement

FODMAP is an acronym for fermentable; oligosaccharides (e.g., fructans and galactans); disaccharides (e.g., lactose); monosaccharides (e.g., excess fructose); and polyols (e.g., sorbitol, mannitol, maltitol, xylitol, and isomalt), essentially short-chain carbohydrates. In plain English, this means the list of foods to avoid includes fermented foods, many fruits and vegetables, as well as dairy, wheat, and rye. Here's what happens if FODMAP is an issue for you: In most people, these foods are digested in the small intestine. When they are not, they pass, mostly undigested, into the large intestine, where the bacteria feast on them producing a lot of gas and changes in gut movement. If the gut empties too quickly, you get diarrhea; if it's too slow, constipation takes place. Either way, you know something is not right. In 1999, Dr. Sue Shepherd, a dietitian in Australia, identified the problem foods (mostly sugars and insoluble fiber) and created a new diet, the low-FODMAP diet, based on avoiding these particular foods.

In a recent study in the journal *Gastroenterology*, researchers followed several adults who said they have gluten sensitivity and were confirmed not to have celiac disease. The researchers discovered that gastrointestinal symptoms improved significantly in 34 of 37 patients if they reduced their FODMAP intake. Just three participants showed improvement when following only a gluten-free diet.

As if the gluten-free diet wasn't daunting enough, the low-FODMAP diet can seem completely overwhelming. Fortunately, Sue Shepherd has several books available on the subject, including cookbooks. Here's a list of foods by group that need to be avoided. You'll notice some overlap with the gluten-free diet, as wheat and rye are also among foods to avoid in the low-FODMAP diet.

- **Fructose:** honey, apple, mango, pear, watermelon, and high-fructose corn syrup
- **Fructans:** artichoke, (globe and Jerusalem), asparagus, beet, chicory, dandelion leaves, garlic (in large amounts), leek, onion, radicchio, lettuce, spring onion, wheat, rye, and inulin
- **Lactose:** milk, ice cream, custard, dairy desserts, condensed and evaporated milk, milk powder, yogurt, margarine, and soft, unripened cheeses
- **Galacto-oligosaccharides (GOS):** legumes, such as kidney beans and chickpeas
- **Polyols:** apple, apricot, avocado, cherries, nectarine, pear, plum, prune, and mushrooms. The artificial sweeteners sorbitol, mannitol, xylitol, maltitol, and isomalt are also in this group.

Shepherd says that onions are the number one culprit and avoiding these, alone, will make a big difference. Patients, usually with the help of a dietitian, will eliminate all of these foods for a brief period of time (a few weeks) and then add back one group at a time, observing any changes in reaction to each group.

In addition, if you are a gum chewer, try eliminating gum, too. Sugar-free gums include one of the artificial sweeteners, such as maltitol, xylitol, or sorbitol.

Breath tests for lactose and fructose are available. Taking these tests will help you know whether you need to eliminate or can keep these entire groups of foods in your diet.

Wheat Allergy

Wheat allergy may seem like it's another side of celiac disease, but it is very different. Whereas celiac disease is an autoimmune disorder, wheat allergy is an immune disorder. Depending on the route of exposure to wheat, it can manifest itself as classic food allergy affecting the skin, gastrointestinal tract, or respiratory tract; wheat-dependent, exercise-induced allergic reaction; occupational asthma (baker's asthma) and rhinitis; or hives.

Extreme cases can lead to a life-threatening reaction. Swelling or tightness in the throat, difficulty breathing or swallowing, dizziness or fainting, pale blue skin color, and fast heart rate are indications of a reaction that requires immediate emergency care.

Ways Wheat Allergy Differs from Celiac Disease

- It is an immune rather than an autoimmune disorder.
- Unlike celiac disease, wheat allergy is more prevalent in children and can be outgrown.
- Wheat allergies are treated by removing wheat from the diet, but some forms of wheat, such as spelt, einkorn, kamut, and farro, may still be tolerated.
- Wheat and gluten are not the same thing; although all wheat contains gluten, not all gluten comes from wheat.
- Depending on the severity of symptoms, some people can eat small amounts of wheat.
- Allergy shots can help relieve symptoms in some wheat-allergic patients.
- Unlike celiac disease in which symptoms can occur minutes, hours, or even days after eating gluten, an allergic reaction to wheat will likely happen within minutes or a few hours after ingestion.

Testing for Wheat Allergy

Immuno-allergy tests for IgE antibodies and skin prick tests are used in diagnosis. Maintaining an elimination diet and keeping a food diary may help with this diagnosis.

Wheat allergies are treated by removing wheat products from the diet. Depending on how the allergy is expressed, the doctor may recommend avoiding skin care products, lotions, and soaps that contain wheat or wheat germ oil.

Who Can Diagnose Me?

An allergist or a naturopathic physician can run the tests to help determine whether you have a wheat allergy. A dietitian or naturopathic doctor can help you establish a regimen to eliminate wheat from your diet and from the products you use.

Other Conditions That Might Benefit from a Gluten-free Diet

Although there's little scientific evidence to recommend avoiding gluten for these conditions, many people that have them report a benefit from the gluten-free diet.

- Autism spectrum disorder
- Attention deficit/hyperactivity disorder
- Multiple sclerosis
- Irritable bowel syndrome
- Rheumatoid arthritis

Raising Your GF IQ: Common Questions About Other Conditions and Gluten

Is there a link between gluten and autism?

For years parents with children on the autism spectrum disorder (ASD) have put their children on a gluten-free/casein-free diet with varying degrees of success. But scientists, including those in a 2010 study from the University of Rochester, concluded that eliminating gluten and casein from the diet of children with autism had no impact on their behavior, sleep, or bowel patterns.

Now, a study from researchers at Columbia University Medical Center in June 2013 is the first to show that some children with autism appear to have increased immune sensitivity to gluten in a way that is different from celiac disease. More research is needed, but as researchers are also developing biomarkers for gluten sensitivity, look for more on this subject.[4]

Can I control my thyroid disease by cutting out gluten?

There is some evidence that if you have celiac disease and you are diagnosed early, you reduce your risk of acquiring other autoimmune diseases. The autoimmune thyroid disease Hashimoto's disease, a form of hypothyroidism or low thyroid function, is in that category, as is Grave's disease, the autoimmune form of hyperthyroidism, the production of too much thyroid hormone.

Eliminating gluten if you don't have celiac disease will not regulate your thyroid function, in any case, and should not be used as a treatment for thyroid conditions. Only a medical professional can sort out these conditions and treat you for the correct ailment.

Can I prevent diabetes if I go gluten-free?

Some medical experts think that diagnosing celiac disease in young children can prevent or delay the onset of type 1 diabetes, the autoimmune disease. For one thing, they share common genes (HLA-DQ2 and HLA-DQ8) and 5 to 10 percent of people with type 1 diabetes also have celiac disease. Researchers are studying the relationship of the two diseases.

But type 1 diabetes, which is seen most frequently in children, is often diagnosed first. Because the percentage is significant and the genetic predisposition is known, physicians recommend testing children for celiac disease once they've had the diagnosis of type 1 diabetes.

The challenge of maintaining both a diabetic and GFD can be stressful at first since the diabetic diet focuses on complex carbs that digest slowly and many gluten-free options rely on simple carbs that metabolize quickly. Finding that balance can be tricky. However, getting the GFD under control makes it much easier to control blood sugar and insulin levels.

Going on a gluten-free diet if you do not have celiac disease will probably not be of any benefit in preventing type 1 diabetes.

Type 2 diabetes is a different medical condition whereby either the body does not produce enough insulin or the cells ignore the insulin. It is the most common form of diabetes, and weight and age enter into the equation. Eating a gluten-free diet won't help in treating this condition. In fact, if you trade gluten for gluten-free products, you'll be eating more calories and less beneficial whole grains, exactly the opposite of what is recommended for patients with type 2 diabetes.

Interestingly, the rate of cardiovascular disease, metabolic syndrome, and type 2 diabetes is lower in people with celiac disease, according to researchers from Beth Israel Deaconess Medical Center (BIDMC).[5]

My doctor says I might have leaky gut. What is it and why should I worry?

Leaky gut is not a true medical term that's recognized by most traditional physicians. Nevertheless, some alternative practitioners use the term when they refer to increased intestinal permeability or damage to the intestinal lining. It's a reference to incompletely digested proteins and fats and waste that would normally be absorbed in the intestines, which instead is leaking into the bloodstream. This can cause bloating, excessive gas, fatigue, food sensitivities, joint pain, skin rashes, and more. It can be caused by a number of conditions, including gluten sensitivity or celiac disease, which should be ruled out by a gastroenterologist before attempting to eliminate such foods as gluten from the diet.

4

How to Pick a Physician and Get on the Road to Proper Treatment

As a friend posted on Facebook, picking a doctor is "like shopping for anything. Check the fit, the value. You are the consumer, the customer. If your doctor doesn't get that, find another doctor."

If finding the perfect doctor was as easy as going to an online dating service, we'd all be set. But finding the right doc isn't that simple. Treating a gluten issue and related health concerns isn't like setting a broken bone. You need someone who is willing to be your long-term partner for good health; someone who is a good diagnostician, but is also a bit holistic; a colleague; and a friend. It is not always beneficial or necessary to have an up-close-and-personal relationship with your health-care provider. A comfort level, yes.

You'll be seeing more than one doc: your regular primary care physician can screen you through blood tests and, if the blood serology is positive, will refer you to a gastroenterologist who will perform a small bowel endoscopy to confirm the diagnosis. You and your primary care physician and gastroenterologist will discuss further related testing for nutrient deficiencies, bone density, and such. Following are some tips to help you get diagnosed.

(If you have DH, you might also have a dermatologist on your team; for gluten ataxia or neuropathy, a neurologist may be called in, too.)

Check This Out:
Things to Ask Your Insurance Provider
Before You Get Tested

- Which celiac tests will you cover?
- Will you pay for endoscopy?
- Will you cover bone density studies and how frequently can I be tested?
- Do you cover visits to a dietitian? How many?
- Do you pay for genetic testing?

Affordable Care Act ("Obamacare")

Will the Affordable Care Act (ACA) make life easier or more difficult for people with celiac disease? Probably a little of both. As of this writing, the Affordable Care Act is just being implemented.

Under ACA, no one can be turned down for health-care coverage based on a preexisting condition and you cannot be charged a higher rate for coverage. (However, you might need to change plans or providers to receive coverage.)

On the other hand, "All the reasons that people avoid going to doctors because they won't be covered, go away," says Andrea Levario, executive director of the American Celiac Disease Alliance, an advocacy organization that represents the needs of patients with celiac disease and other gluten-related conditions. "They will be covered and I expect more people will be diagnosed as a result," says Levario.

Standard benefits will probably vary by health exchange. Before selecting a plan that is right for you, you'll want to ask about the coverage for diagnosing and treating celiac disease as well as genetic testing and follow-up tests for family members. For more information, go to healthcare.gov.

Communicating with
Your Doctor About Your Symptoms

Patients tend not to tell their doctor how badly they are feeling unless the doctor asks.

—Dr. Robert G. Schwartz, gastroenterologist

Sure, you have good days and bad days. Your symptoms are vague and you could fill a notebook with them. How do you convince your doctor you are not being a drama queen (or king) and that you may have this serious autoimmune disease.

For one thing, quit whining. I mean that in a nice way. Unburdening yourself in the doctor's office can make it difficult for a diagnostician to sort through your misery and get to the symptoms.

I asked Dr. Schwartz, who is both a celiac patient and a gastroenterologist, what he thinks is an effective way to communicate with your doctor. Here are some of his tips:

Be as concrete as possible. When you visit a doctor, it's difficult to explain all your symptoms, especially since many adults don't really have specific digestive symptoms. Imagine you have ten minutes. You have to let him or her know if something is impacting or limiting your quality of life without falling into the trap of, "When I eat pasta, it doesn't agree with me." Patients sometimes say, "I tend to burp a lot." But burping can be a symptom related to anxiety and the doctor might want to send you to a psychiatrist. Outline what is making your life difficult to manage. A doctor will take notice if you say, "I'm tired all the time; I have terrible stomach pains every time I eat; I get awful headaches; I'm in the bathroom so much I can't leave the house; I have to call in sick at least once a week." Don't make these up, but imagine why you are there and what you need help with, he advises. As much as that whole wheat pasta with marinara sauce was outrageous until it made you throw up, stick to the overarching concerns.

Make a list. Include what's been bothering you, in as much useful detail as possible. Dr. Schwartz also suggests asking the doctor to run a panel of tests that includes checking for anemia, thyroid function, and celiac disease. Depending on the insurance carrier, he does say that you might have to pay for some of these tests out of pocket. Selecting a doctor who is knowledgeable about celiac disease will increase your chances for getting the diagnostic tests paid for by your insurance plan, as he or she probably knows the proper justifications and insurance codes for specific tests and how often these tests can be run. This is especially important if your insurance carrier requires preauthorization for tests and procedures.

Make a List of Your Symptoms

The first thing to do is to sort through questions and concerns before going to your own doctors. That is important. Digressing into personal stories sends the discussion in a different direction and you might leave the office wondering what your visit accomplished.

Lists are handy even if they are scratched out on a napkin. They create a reminder and establish an agenda. You only have a certain amount of time for your appointment. Even if you begin yakking, because ultimately you will want to pick a friendly, knowledgeable physician, you'll both know there's a game plan. Before the appointment is over, your doctor should say, "What else is on your list?" If not, you have it in front of you so you can remind him or her.

If you are having a procedure that requires sedation (say, a colonoscopy or an endoscopy) and you have questions, write a note and ask your doc to give the answer to your spouse or whoever's picking you up, or bring along a health proxy to take notes for you.

Questions to Ask a Physician Once You Have Been Diagnosed with CD, DH, or GS

Yes, more questions. Once you have a diagnosis, you will quickly move from the world of ill health to a world of good health and maintaining that good health means following up on issues that keep you in the pink. Here are some things you'll want to know:

- What additional tests do I need to have done?
- And you might as well ask: Should others in my family be tested and how do I do that?
- Will any of my medications need to be adjusted once my celiac disease is under control?
- Should I take vitamins? Which ones?
- Should I take a probiotic? Which one?
- How do I find out if my medications are gluten-free?
- Do I need any special inoculations? Should I have the shingles vaccine; the pneumococcal pneumonia vaccine?
- What should I expect from a follow-up visit and when do you need to see me again?
- Once I'm healed, how often should I come back to see you?
- Can my primary care physician follow me if I don't have any other issues?
- Should I have a bone density test? How frequently should I have it done?
- Who can help me find out what I can eat? Should I see a dietitian? Which ones specialize in gluten-free diets?

The Final Word

Pick a doctor who knows about digestive issues, celiac disease, and gluten sensitivity. Be assertive but not whiny. Restate the obvious. "I need your help to sort this out. I am housebound by constant bouts of diarrhea. My food goes right through me and it's affecting my quality of life." Be persistent and firm. Don't let someone tell you nothing is wrong if you believe otherwise.

The Doctor Who Diagnoses Might Not Be the Doctor You See Forever

At first, you will be driven by symptoms. Someone needs to figure out what's eating you, why you throw up three times a week, why your brain is

Gut Instincts:
Finding the Best Doc Might Require a Second Opinion

One patient's definition of a good doctor might be totally different than another's. Some of it may depend on your personal health needs and insurance coverage, as well as the physician's personality. But more important, this is truly a topic for which you need to go with your gut. You need to feel confident that your doctor is interested, concerned, and thorough.

I posed the question of how to find the right doctor to my Facebook friends and several support group leaders to see what they do and what they recommend to others. Besides, this is a topic where it's always good to have a second opinion. Here are some of their suggestions:

- Ask your primary care doctor who he or she recommends to treat celiac disease.
- Do some online research, searching for doctors in your area who specialize in celiac disease. It's a good way to check credentials and see whether there is anything alarming in the doctor's record.
- Post a request for recommendations on the Celiac Listserv (to subscribe, see page 303).
- Check with a local support group. Ask its medical adviser. (One support group leader interviewed a doctor to be the group's medical adviser, checked his background, and ended up using him herself.)
- Do a search on the Internet. Sometimes you will find reviews from other patients.
- Check with a local medical school or medical center, Some have a celiac center or doctors specializing in the disease.

You can rely on Match.com to check for compatible astrology signs and temperament, but that's not going to help you find a doctor who is easy to talk to. However, you can attend a lecture given by that physician. Support groups and hospital community education programs frequently invite physicians to speak. It's a good bet that the physician welcomes new patients if he or she is giving a lecture. After the program, talk to the doctor. Ask if he or she treats other patients with celiac disease.

foggy like you have early-onset Alzheimer's disease. We all want to understand what is happening and how we can get off the treadmill of symptoms that are interfering with life.

Sorting through this laundry list of ailments might take a specialist in celiac disease or gluten sensitivity. But once you have the diagnosis and have to ask, "What's next?" You might need a referral to another doctor who will become your friend for life, literally.

Why Consulting a Dietitian Might be Good for Your Health

By now, you've probably guessed that staying on a GFD is no gluten-free cakewalk (see "Diet Diligence," page 82). First you need to understand what you can and cannot have, make certain you can eat safely wherever you go, and finally, be willing to follow that regimen. The American College of Gastroenterology, the American Academy of Nutrition and Dietetics, and many leading patient groups recommend adding a registered dietitian (RD) to your health-care team to help you follow the gluten-free regimen.

But not every dietitian is qualified and knowledgeable about the GFD. Look for an RD who has additional certifications in areas of practice such as celiac disease. In addition, many physician practices, local celiac support groups, celiac medical centers, and children's hospitals have knowledgeable RDs on staff or a list of dietitians they recommend.

Because counseling from a nutrition professional is deemed to be "necessary and the standard of care for patients with celiac disease," most insurance providers will cover visits to a dietitian if celiac disease is listed as the reason (another reason to get tested and to get a proper diagnosis). Although the same RDs will be helpful to patients with gluten sensitivity, insurance companies are not likely to cover these visits for this new subsection, as yet.

It's Okay to Fire Your Doctor

There are creeps in every profession. If the physician tries to dismiss you and your symptoms or refers you to a psychiatrist when you know you are having very real physical issues, ditch him or her quickly and find another physician. And what if you want to see another physician in the same practice? If you feel uncomfortable, you may want to switch to another practice. However, the likelihood of running into your former doctor in the same practice is not high. But to play it safe, confide in one of the office staff and find out which days your original physician is in the operating room or in another office, so you can schedule visits when you are guaranteed not to cross paths.

The Rock Stars in Research

Several hospitals around the United States have a center for digestive diseases, and specifically one that specializes in celiac disease, gluten sensitivity, and related disorders. You'll find a list of those centers in Resources, page 305. The heads of these organizations are the stars of the digestive disease world. Many are mentioned in the pages of this book.

These folks do research, speak to medical and patient groups, and see patients. They are the experts, but do you need to see one of them to diagnose you? In a word, no. For the most part, your diagnosis will hopefully be "by the book." So why am I telling you about the medical rock stars? If you have complications, such as a condition that does not improve on the gluten-free diet, inconclusive test results, or other worrisome secondary conditions, you'll want an expert to weigh in on your case. That doesn't happen too often, thankfully. But it's nice to know about these folks in case you need their help. They are more than generous with their time and you can make an appointment with one of them or a colleague in that practice. You might need to obtain a referral from your primary care physician to be covered by your insurance.

The other reason you should know about them is because they are doing the bulk of the research in celiac disease, gluten sensitivity, and related conditions. While you might not understand all the medical papers they write, staying abreast of the latest medical breakthroughs is important to your health.

And here's one more reason. Medicine is usually joined at the hip with the pharmaceutical industry that provides a lot of money for medical research. (Okay, don't tell anyone I said that.) But there is no medicine for celiac disease, just a gluten-free diet. So the money for research is difficult to come by. And ask any researcher about applying for grants. Grant money is tight and the competition is fierce.

Individual contributions help more than you can imagine. If you can donate to one of these centers, please do so. It's an investment in your future. Each center's website has a Donate button displayed prominently. They are not shy about asking.

Too bad some of these rock stars can't team up with Bruce Springsteen, Lady Gaga, or One Direction. A concert in Madison Square Garden with one of them would fund a lot of research. But these folks are more excited about mucosal variations/anomalies than fancy guitars, and we should all be grateful for that.

The Diet's the Medicine (for Now)

Unfortunately, there is no medication or pill for CD, or gluten sensitivity, for that matter; the gluten-free diet is all that is available at the moment. But you are not alone in thinking that managing your health through constant dietary vigilance is sometimes downright impossible. Researchers estimate that a large number of people with celiac disease are not sticking to the diet. This chapter delves into some of the more interesting things on the horizon for anyone with a gluten-related disorder.

The Future of Treatment

Researchers at the University of Chicago Celiac Disease Center are in hopes of discovering a cure for celiac disease by 2026. A change in the URL for its website reflects that goal: www.cureceliacdisease.org. In the more immediate future, at least three drugs and one vaccine are in the development stage to help people manage the gluten-free diet. It will be a race to the finish or should I say, to the FDA, where final approval is needed. (Unfortunately, none of these will treat symptoms of gluten sensitivity or wheat allergy. If you have gluten sensitivity, fear not. Medical experts are breaking ground in other areas in which gluten affects us and gluten sensitivity is a top priority.)

Meanwhile researchers and drug developers are vying to have the first approved product to treat celiac disease. The drugs take different approaches: One is an enzyme designed to break down the gluten protein, one is a vaccine to help desensitize you to gluten, the third is a medication intended to help prevent leaky gut (intestinal permeability), and the fourth actually binds to the gluten molecule to escort it safely from your body.

The drugs are in clinical trials with people who have celiac disease, which means the FDA has given them the green light to move forward. It's likely at least one will be approved in the next five to ten years.

Here's a rundown:

Alvine Pharmaceuticals' ALV003 involves two strong digestive enzymes to help break down the gluten protein before the immune system reacts to it. This medication is to be taken in conjunction with the GFD to protect against eating small amounts of gluten, such as from cross-contamination.

ImmusanT's Nexvax2 uses a vaccine approach that is not unlike allergy shots, exposing the person to small amounts of gluten peptides to help induce the immune system to tolerate gluten. This vaccine works with patients who have the HLA-DQ2 gene, which is about 95 percent of celiac patients.

Alba Therapeutics Corporation's AT-1001 was the first potential celiac disease drug in formulation. AT-1001, now called larazotide acetate, is designed to improve the intestinal barrier, limiting the amount of gluten that can pass through, and would be used along with the GFD to reduce the risk from cross-contamination.

BioLineRx's BL-7010. In this concept, BL-7010 binds to the gluten protein and escorts it through the digestive system, where it is expelled through stool. It could minimize gut damage from cross-contamination, but is not designed for use when eating large amounts of gluten.

It's not clear which of these celiac disease drugs, if any, will make it to market. Nevertheless, this early research may pave the way for future research and more sophisticated medications. And it's good news for all of us. While these treatments focus on ways to prevent gluten from causing an autoimmune response in people with celiac disease, other aspects of that research examine the gluten molecule itself, which is likely to have far-reaching benefits for a larger group of people with gluten issues.

One more item bears watching:

AN-PEP enzyme (prolyl endopeptidase), developed in the Netherlands, may be marketed in the United States by the time this book comes out. Because it is sold as a food supplement, it does not need FDA approval. This enzyme breaks down gluten in the stomach and escorts it safely through the small intestine without causing intestinal damage. Research shows this enzyme has been quite effective in detoxifying gluten to some degree. While it sounds promising for celiacs, do your research and talk to your doctor before you try this.

Don't Wash Your Hands Until You Read This—Germs and All Gluten-Related Disorders

How many times have you heard someone say, "What's up with the big jump in people with celiac disease, gluten issues, or with food allergies in general?" There's no question all of these are on the rise. And no one knows why. But one leading theory points in the direction of friendly bugs that seem to be missing in people with gluten sensitivities and food allergies. Basically, we are just too clean!

In one report, researchers studied a region on the Finnish-Russian border that historically was a single province. The populations are culturally, linguistically, and genetically related. But researchers looking at type 1 diabetes, another autoimmune disease, found that the disease is six times less frequent in the Russian citizens than in their Finnish counterparts. The incidence of autoimmune thyroid disease and allergies was also significantly less. This information was reported in the *New York Times* article "Who has the Guts for Gluten?"[1]

At the time of this research, roughly a decade ago, Russia's per-capita income was one fifteenth of Finland's. Because of cleanliness standards, the Russians were exposed to a greater variety and quantity of microbes, including many that were simply absent in Finland, the article says.

Friendly Flora

Your intestinal flora (bacteria) might play a leading role in what ails you or keeps you healthy, it turns out. Two terms you will be hearing a lot about in the future are *microbiota* and *microbiome*, and both have to do with the friendly bacteria in our body.

The bottom line is that researchers think the Western world has become too clean. We take antibiotics that wipe out the friendly flora; we use hand sanitizers and disinfectants to kill all the germs around us. This reduced exposure to bacterial antigens during the first eighteen months of life causes the immune system development to be skewed toward producing a response to future antigens that leads to higher risk of allergic and autoimmune conditions.

Researchers are documenting this difference in the microbial makeup of people with celiac disease and food allergies. It's too soon to know the role that our bacteria play in these conditions or whether it is possible to manipulate the microbiota to treat food allergy and autoimmune disease. But at the University of Chicago Celiac Center, mice treated with antibiotics were found to have more food allergies than those left untreated. What's more, the researchers identified a type of bacteria living in the colon of healthy mice that was able to correct susceptibility to food allergy when given back to mice with food allergies.

At the moment, most of the research centers around infants and babies who have fewer other health and lifestyle issues planted in their microbiome. Take a look at the discussion about breastfeeding and introducing gluten to infants, on page 33, for more about this exciting work.

Needless to say, the significance of microbial research to people with food allergy, gluten sensitivity, and celiac disease has the medical world abuzz with excitement. An entire initiative called the American Gut Project is taking place, looking at the microbial makeup of thousands of people, as related to their lifestyle and diet, with the notion that this research could unlock the key to many diseases.

Could this be an alternative treatment for infants, children, and adults with celiac disease? Could this be the root cause of gluten sensitivity, too? It's too early to tell. But it's a hot topic in the medical world these days. So when your kids refuse to wash their hands before dinner, they might have something there.[2]

Probiotics

One thing is certain. Adults can repopulate the flora in their intestine to some degree and help aid digestion by adding probiotics to their diet. Defined as friendly bacteria, probiotics help aid digestion and boost the autoimmune system, something that benefits anyone with celiac disease, gluten sensitivity, and other gluten-related issues.

"The presence of bacteria in the GI tract is fundamental to developing a healthy gut immune system," says Dr. Guandalini, MD, professor and section chief, Pediatric Gastroenterology, University of Chicago, and founder and medical director, Celiac Disease Center, where much of the research on the microbiota and celiac disease is taking place in the United States.

Dietary supplements are available in a wide variety of dosages and a wide range of probiotic strains. Finding one that best suits your needs and issues is largely trial and error. Strains that are often recommended include such words as *lactobacillus*, *bifidobacteria*, and *acidophilus*.

In addition, some foods are a great source of probiotics. Think about adding such foods as yogurt (with live cultures), miso, kefir, sauerkraut, pickles, dark chocolate, and kombucha (fermented tea) to your diet.

Raising Your GF IQ:
Frequently Asked Questions About Treatment

Can I desensitize myself by eating a little gluten every day?

No. No. No! Not if you have celiac disease. Your T-cells (responsible for bad things, such as cancer) have finally quieted down now that you've stopped eating gluten. Each exposure puts you at greater risk for developing lymphomas and other digestive cancers as well as other autoimmune diseases. Don't stir up trouble.

In fact, I don't know of any conditions caused by ingesting gluten where this is a helpful technique. Some research is being done to desensitize kids who have severe peanut allergies. But peanut allergy has a completely different physiology than celiac disease.

Can I outgrow this?

In the forties and fifties, physicians thought a child could outgrow celiac disease by removing most foods and adding them back very slowly over many months. I was one of those kids. Now we know that celiac disease is for life.

Research is just beginning on gluten sensitivity so it's too soon to know whether people outgrow this condition. Some people seem to tolerate small amounts of gluten occasionally. And if someone with gluten sensitivity removes all gluten for an extended period of time, it's possible they can return to a gluten-containing diet. Because gluten sensitivity is not autoimmune in nature, trying gluten to see whether you are still reacting might make you feel crappy but it will not cause any long-term damage.

If you are adopting a gluten-free lifestyle by choice, you'll need to monitor your symptoms and your diet based on the reasons you chose this diet. However, people do say they seem much more sensitive to small amounts of gluten once they've removed it from their regimen. You'll have to be the judge of that.

Is the flu shot safe for people with celiac disease?

Yes, physicians recommend the flu shot for all celiac patients. Exclusion criteria are exactly the same as for other people. Unless you have an allergy to eggs, or have a high fever, there is no reason to avoid getting a flu shot. However, to be sure, discuss this with a physician who knows your personal history.

The Skinny on the
Gluten-free Diet and Weight Loss

Welcome to the latest urban myth. Don't be fooled by the word *diet*. Gluten is a health issue for millions of people with celiac disease, gluten sensitivity or wheat allergy. Removing it makes those folks feel a whole lot healthier. But a new version of the Atkins diet, it's not. If you are gluten-free by choice (or avoiding gluten for any reason), pay close attention to fiber and nutrient issues. These are plentiful in wheat products, but gluten-free prepared foods are notoriously void of both.

If You Become a Slave to Fashion, You May Outgrow Your Clothes

> In one way I'm glad that gluten-free has gotten so much attention, but it's kind of gone sideways. There is not the increased level of awareness and diagnosis of celiac disease I was hoping for. Without a solid diagnosis, it is human nature for people to start straying back to gluten, not understanding the danger they may be in if they are celiac. A lot of the increase in popularity of the gluten-free diet is being driven by the public and unfortunately not by doctors being more aware, and diagnosing more people. Some people think wheat is bad for everyone. I don't think that's true, but it is one of the most problematic foods out there.
>
> —CHRISTINE DOHERTY, ND, WHO SPECIALIZES IN
> CELIAC DISEASE AND GLUTEN-RELATED ISSUES

Is there anyone who hasn't given up gluten for one reason or another? It seems that every day, a new celebrity or star athlete announces he or she has gone gluten-free. They feel wonderful and have lost weight. But the biggest misconception about the GFD is that this diet is a way to lose weight. If you decide to stop eating gluten-filled pancakes, pasta, pizza and the like and replace these with gluten-free counterparts, watch out. You can potentially increase your calorie intake by as much as 20 percent and you'll be decreasing your fiber and nutrient intake at the same time.

Here's something to chew on:

- Rice flour is 578 calories per cup; wheat flour is 455 calories per cup.

- Gluten-free English muffins contain 200 calories; gluten-filled English muffins contain 120 calories per serving.
- A gluten-free bagel is 320 calories; a gluten-filled bagel is 240 calories.
- Gluten-free cookies can pack 60 calories per cookie.
- Gluten-free baked goods need extra sugar and fat to make them taste good.
- Rice flour and starches are the go-to flours for gluten-free baking. These are empty calories, absent of fiber and nutrients and high on the glycemic index.
- Wheat flour contains B vitamins, niacin, and fiber. Unless rice flour is fortified, you won't be getting these if you give up gluten. (See "Vitamins and Supplements," page 109.)

As Alice Bast, president of the National Foundation for Celiac Awareness (NFCA), reminds us, "Gluten-free junk food is still junk food."

To lose weight while on a GFD, cut back on those pancakes, cookies, pretzels, and cake and fill up on veggies, fruits, and low-fat protein. Limit your intake of simple carbohydrates, such as white rice flour, starches, and white sugar, which tend to spike blood sugar levels and leave you tired and hungry again in no time. Pick nutritionally dense gluten-free whole grains and flours (chickpea, quinoa, millet, amaranth, buckwheat, and sorghum) that digest more slowly, keeping blood sugar levels more stable. Try replacing 50 percent of the fat in your recipes with an equal amount of unsweetened applesauce, pureed white beans (yes, really!), or mashed banana. Not only are you reducing the fat in baked goods, but you are also increasing the nutritional profile of your recipes. Watch your total calorie intake, avoid processed foods, and don't forget to exercise.

It's clear that total calorie intake from any source is critical, because more calories can lead to weight gain, which can lead to metabolic syndrome and increased risk of type 2 diabetes, heart disease, and stroke. Because this gluten-free diet is in our hands and we cook a lot from scratch, we get to drive what goes into our mouth.

Take a Mediterranean Cruise . . . Through the Grocery Aisles

A study in the February 2013 *New England Journal of Medicine*, saw a 30 percent improvement in the health of 7,500 people taking part in a Mediterranean diet study.

Don't you want what they are eating? Well, you can have it. A diet full of veggies, fruit, olive oil, nuts, and wine—hey, it's healthy *and* it's all gluten-free. Add fish, chicken, and turkey, and you are basically eating from the outside aisles of the supermarket, where the food is healthy and not processed.

Is this all sounding familiar? The Mediterranean diet and the gluten-free diet have a lot in common. Both would have you eating from the outside aisles and eating minimally processed foods.

Speaking of diet, the next section is devoted to just that.

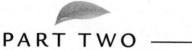

—— PART TWO ——

Diet
When Food Is the Medicine

Have you noticed that gluten-free is everywhere? A Quest Diagnostics ad runs every night on my television—little frowny green faces bounce around the screen as a narrator reminds us there are many symptoms for celiac disease, but one test to diagnose it. A well-known television celebrity chef shows off her lasagna recipes for snowy days and one is gluten-free.

Life is good in the kingdom of the gluten-free, but I think back to when my son, Jeremy, was growing up in the nineties. Even ordering a burger at McDonald's was a challenge. "Hamburger, pickle, ketchup, tomato, mustard, and hold the bun," he'd say. The employee would look at my ten-year-old as if he had just grown another head. I felt badly. But explaining our diet and defending our gluten-free needs was all part of the drill.

Today everyone gets it. A gluten frenzy of sorts is taking place, and it's synonymous with abundance, understanding, and choices. Grocery store shelves are filled to overflowing with products labeled "gluten-free." And it's easier than ever to find safe gluten-free foods, thanks to two food-labeling rules—one of exclusion that warns when a product contains wheat (FALCPA, see page 117) and one of inclusion that lets consumers know when a product is gluten-free (FDA gluten-free food label rule, see page 118). With so much information and so many safe products, you might be asking why I devote so many pages to the gluten-free diet. Isn't this all the information you need to live well?

Not exactly. There's a huge gray area in between safe and not safe, where products are questionable and ingredients may be hidden. Then there's the entire subject of gluten in medications, lotions, and booze. And these nuanced details make the difference between surviving and thriving.

This section will answer all your questions about making safe choices and knowing where gluten might lurk in foods and where cross-contamination can occur. It includes sections on foods that can trip you up and foods that pack a nutritious whole-grain (gluten-free) punch.

This is not a "diet" diet section, however. It's doubtful you can lose weight by switching from gluten to gluten-free. A gluten-free diet filled with prepared foods can be calorie-laden and downright unhealthy. In fact, it can be higher in calories and glycemic load. Junk food is junk food, carbs are carbs, and calories are calories—gluten-free or not.

What about sharing a kitchen with gluten-eaters? You'll find helpful tips for setting up your own kitchen and ways to avoid cross-contamination at home. Is easy meal planning sounding impossible right about now? You'll find tips for that, too. And finally, you'll find fifteen of my favorite recipes for foods I never thought I'd have again—safe for you and delicious for everyone.

So, don't run away just yet. If gluten-free is part of your life, this portion of the book is the blueprint for your future, your life without gluten.

Gut Reaction:
Forty Years in a Gluten-free Desert

Early on, the gluten-free food I ate tasted much like munching on sand. Okay, I really don't know much about sand and how it tastes, but everything I ate was so dry, crumbly, and flavorless, it might as well have been sand. I decided to stick to a naturally gluten-free diet of meats, fruit, and vegetables.

The information was sparse and I was constantly dodging misinformation. At various times I was told: avoid alcohol, vinegar, oats, natural and artificial flavors; eat Corn Flakes or have Rice Krispies. I ate the two breakfast cereals and avoided the other items on this list for years, not realizing that Corn Flakes and Rice Krispies contained malt (from barley—most definitely gluteny), whereas vinegar, many flavoring, and most alcohols are safe. I had it totally backward. (Today there's even a gluten-free version of Rice Krispies.)

What's more, the term *cross-contamination*, and its implications for celiac patients, was not known.

These days the gluten-free foods are plentiful and the choices are amazing, from delicious bagels to toaster pastries, from good pasta to gluten-free pies, cookies by the dozen, and delicious-tasting breads. Thanks to a wide assortment of ingredients and great cookbooks, baking is easier, too, letting me have more control over what I eat and helping me avoid some of the unhealthy processed products, except as treats. I feel like my exodus is over and I can now eat more safely and enjoy a feast of riches.

Gluten 101

What Exactly Is It?

It sounds like a simple question; so, how does this diet get so complicated? Just as celiac disease is the great impersonator that can fool even the most astute physician, gluten, too, wears many disguises that can trip up even the savviest celiac or gluten avoider. Ever notice that *glue* and *gluten* sound similar? It's no coincidence. *Gluten* means "glue" in Latin and gluten is a sticky protein that holds things together. For example, it's a bond that creates elasticity in pizza. As a baker, I often suffer gluten envy, wishing I could have some of this gorgeous elasticity in my own baked goods.

Explaining Gluten

First of all, for all you Dr. Science fans, here's a quick look at the gluten molecule, broken down:

Gluten is not one substance but a complex substance made up of many proteins and some fats. Most of the proteins are prolamins, which cereal grains use to store energy in their seeds. Literally hundreds of different prolamins found in wheat gluten (many more in rye and barley) contain amino acid sequences capable of triggering an immune response.

An analysis of wheat prolamins further divides them into two groups: gliadins and glutenins. Gliadins are a primary cause of celiac disease.

Glutenins are usually harmless, but each patient varies in sensitivity to different proteins.[1]

In short: If you have celiac disease, DH, gluten sensitivity, or wheat allergy, gluten is the stuff you absolutely need to eliminate from your diet (or wheat, if you are wheat-allergic). If you are gluten-free by choice, you have, most likely, made a conscious decision to improve some aspect of your health by avoiding gluten. This essential information will help you as well. Let's talk about managing the diet, avoiding pesky hidden gluten, and which good foods you can enjoy.

Diet Diligence: What You Can and Can't Have

There's a lot of confusion about what you can and can't have. Let's start with the bad news.

Grains to Avoid

- Wheat and all its other forms
  - Durum
  - Einkorn
  - Farina
  - Farro
  - Freekeh
  - Fregola
  - Graham flour
  - Kamut
  - Low-gluten wheat
  - Semolina
  - Spelt
  - Triticale (a cross-breed of wheat and rye)
  - Wheat starch (unless it tests below 20 ppm; see the gluten-free food labeling rule on page 118)
- Rye (not usually disguised in any other forms)
- Barley, also brewer's yeast, and barley malt (Malt from gluten-free grains, such as corn, is okay but infrequently used.)

What You Can Have: The Good Grains

The GFD is more than just rice and rice flour. While these are the go-to favorites, there's a long list of grains that are safe and many are high in nutrients and fiber, too. For information on using all these flours, see page 161.

- Amaranth*
- Buckwheat*
- Corn (corn flour, cornmeal, cornstarch, grits, hominy, masa harina)
- Legume (bean) flours (chickpea, fava bean, navy bean)*
- Millet*
- Nut flours (almond, pecan, hazelnut)*
- Oats (certified gluten-free)*
- Potato (potato flour, potato starch)
- Quinoa*
- Rice (brown rice, white rice, sweet rice)
- Sorghum*
- Tapioca starch
- Teff*

*In their whole-grain form, these are healthy choices for breakfast and pilafs. The flours are good choices to add to baking blends.

Surprising Places Where Gluten Can Lurk

Watch out for gluten (wheat, rye, or barley) in these. If the product contains wheat, it will be noted, but you might not think to read the label unless you know these can be unsafe.

- Barbecue sauce (soy sauce or thickeners)
- Barley beta glucan (barley)
- Bread crumbs (unless labeled "gluten-free")
- Brewer's yeast (from barley)
- Broth/stock/bouillon (can contain wheat gluten or hydrolyzed wheat protein)

- Chocolate chips (occasionally sweetened with barley malt)
- Communion wafers (made with wheat; see page 134)
- Cooking sprays (some contain wheat)
- Couscous (wheat)
- Corn tortillas (can be made on shared equipment with flour tortillas or contain a little added flour for durability)
- Curry paste (may contain wheat)
- Deli meats (a few contain gluten, especially "pressed" meats); see page 136
  - Hamburgers, chicken, and tuna salad (may contain bread or cracker crumbs)
  - Sausages and hot dogs (may contain fillers, soy sauce, or liquid smoke)
- Farina (from semolina; that's wheat!)
- French fries (often coated with flour so flavorings will adhere)
- Licorice (contains wheat, unless specifically labeled "gluten-free")
- Lentils (possible cross-contamination in some processing plants); pick "gluten-free" lentils
- Lipstick and lip gloss (may contain wheat germ oil or wheat)
- Liquid smoke (some contain barley)
- Marinades (may contain soy sauce)
- Matzo and matzo meal
- Medications (some may use undisclosed sources of starch); see page 101
- Miso (often from rice or soy, but can be fermented with rye or barley)
- Mouthwash and toothpaste (usually safe, but occasionally contain wheat)
- Oats (see page 91 for more on gluten-free sources of oats); pick "gluten-free" oats
- Oat beta glucan (oats)
- Oat fiber (not from a safe source of gluten-free oats, unless specified)
- Orzo (wheat)
- Panko (bread crumbs)
- Quinoa (possible cross-contamination in packaging facilities); pick "gluten-free" quinoa

- Salad dressings (may contain soy sauce or thickeners)
- Seasoned rice mixes (wheat may be in the flavoring packet)
- Self-basting poultry (may contain soy sauce or wheat)
- Shredded cheese (flavored cheeses may use flour to hold flavor on the cheese)
- Soy sauce (Most are fermented with wheat. Fermentation does not remove the gluten.) Wheat-free soy sauce and tamari products are available from several companies (see pantry list, page 312).
- Specialty coffee drinks (some contain natural flavorings derived from barley)
- Spice blends and seasonings (occasionally use flour as a carrier agent)
- Stuffing (unless labeled "gluten-free")
- Surimi/imitation crab (some brands contain wheat)
- Teriyaki sauce (contains soy sauce, fermented wheat)
- Teas (barley is sometimes added; tea bags can be sealed with wheat starch)
- Tomato paste (flavored products may contain wheat)
- Vitamins and supplements (check the binding ingredients)
- Worcestershire sauce (some contain gluten)

Some Foods That Sound Dangerous but Are Really Safe

- Artificial flavors*
- Breadfruit
- Buckwheat
- Caramel
- Corn gluten
- Glucose
- Glutinous rice
- Maltodextrin (it's corn-based)
- Monosodium glutamate (MSG)
- Mushrooms (which contain glutamate)
- Mustard flour
- Rice syrup (unless it's from barley malt)
- Yeast

*Artificial flavors are derived from chemicals. You may want to avoid them for other reasons, but unlike natural flavors, they will not contain wheat or barley. (Flavors are rarely derived from rye.)

Gluten-free and wheat-free are not the same. If you have a wheat allergy, you can probably have rye, barley, and perhaps even some forms of ancient wheat, such as spelt and kamut. If you are gluten-free (celiac, DH, gluten ataxia, or gluten-sensitive), all forms of gluten are off the table. If you are gluten-free by choice, the choice is yours—avoid the obvious sources of gluten or dig deeper and eliminate all the sneaky sources, too.

Label Diligence: Ingredients to Avoid

As you probably noted while reading these lists, a lot of products can contain gluten—but the labels may not let you know that. Gluten hides in many ingredients and it doesn't always jump out at you in the supermarket when you are reading labels. Here are some more ways it can appear on labels.

Hydrolyzed Plant Protein

This is used as flavor and texture enhancers in many processed foods. Two of the most popular are derived from wheat or soy. Both will be identified on the food label, as they are among the eight allergens that must be declared under the FALCPA (Food Allergen Labeling and Consumer Protection Act of 2004). Hydrolyzed plant protein is most often from soy, which is gluten-free. (Note that soy sauce is not often gluten-free, because it is often fermented with wheat). Some people have an additional sensitivity to soy products.

Malt

Most often listed as "barley malt," "malt (barley)," "malt flavoring," or "malt extract," malt is created using germinated cereal grains that have been dried in a process known as "malting." Malting converts starches into sugars and is often added as a sweetener in cereals. It can come from rye or wheat, or from corn, rice, quinoa, millet, or sorghum, and its origin is not always stated. If the label says "malt," then you have to dig further.

Steer clear of all of these barley-based foods and ingredients: malted milk, malted milk balls, malted shakes, diastatic malt (usually used in bread making), malted milk ice cream, malt vinegar, and Horlicks and Ovaltine (malt beverages). Single malt liquor is safe as the gluten is removed during the distillation process (see more on alcoholic beverages on page 97).

Wheat Gluten

This ingredient is often used for flavoring, texture, or thickening. It's sometimes added to prepared chicken broth and used as a vegan meat substitute, also known as seitan. Vital wheat gluten (not vital to us!) is a baker's ingredient used in yeast breads.

Gluten Disguised

"I thought I was good with the diet, careful about what I ate, and all that. But every morning around ten a.m. I started to get a headache and kind of bloated. At first it was a vague feeling, but I had it every single day. Then I discovered that my toothpaste contained wheat. I never realized that little bit could be such a big deal."

—A GLUTEN-FREE BLOGGER

Snacks (and Crafts): Kid Things to Avoid

When it comes to kids, you need to watch out for not only snacks, but crafts, too (Play-Doh? Yep, gluteny). Young children like to put everything from candy to clay in their mouths. If you have a child who needs a GFD, you'll want to watch out for these kid-centric crafts and snacks that are often loaded with gluten opportunities.

- Candy (some, such as licorice, Kit Kats, and Milky Way bars, contain wheat)
- Drinks (energy drinks; flavored milk mixes, such as Ovaltine; and specialty coffee drinks that you might be tempted to share with your child can contain wheat or barley)
- Finger paints (may contain wheat)

- French fries (often coated with flour and usually fried in shared equipment)
- Graham crackers (graham is really a form of wheat)
- Modeling clay (many brands contains wheat)
- Papier-mâché (contains wheat)
- Paste/glue (often contains wheat)
- Play-Doh (contains wheat); Mama K's Play Clay is a safe alternative.
- Potato chips (Not all are gluten-free. Pringles products contain wheat, as do many flavored chips.)

Cross-Contamination

How Much Gluten Can I Have?

If you have celiac disease, DH, or gluten ataxia, you should not be asking that question. You need to be on a strict GFD; no cheating allowed. Remember that symptoms vary from person to person. If you feel well, the only way you may know that you are getting gluten in your diet is through periodic blood tests.

If you are gluten sensitive, you will be the best gauge of how much gluten your body can handle. Symptoms led you to this diagnosis and symptoms will let you know when you've gone too far. But most people I know who are gluten-sensitive follow a strict GFD, just like people with celiac disease. The same is true for people who are gluten-free by choice. The reason you have chosen this lifestyle (to fight off inflammation, lose weight, or possibly prevent dementia, for example) is the reason you will want to be vigilant about maintaining it.

What Does "20 Parts per Million" Mean?

In a perfect world, a strict GFD would mean 100 percent gluten-free. But it's not possible to achieve because there is no test for zero gluten. Fortunately, the body cannot detect minute particles of gluten, although sensitivity varies from person to person. A study conducted by Dr. Catassi and Dr. Fasano determined that most people with celiac disease could tolerate

20 ppm of gluten without suffering any harm. That study became known as the "threshold study" and was used by the FDA to establish the less than 20 ppm standard for labeling products as gluten-free.[2]

So what does 20 ppm of gluten mean? That's twenty pennies in $10,000 or twenty minutes in two years. It means 0.002 percent of 20 milligrams of gluten per kilogram of food. You'd have to eat roughly 5 pounds of gluten-free food (at less than 20 ppm) per day for damage to occur, says a statement in the ICDS *Fast Facts*, published by the Celiac Disease Foundation. Products containing less than 20 ppm of gluten are allowed to be labeled "gluten-free" under the FDA gluten-free rule released in August 2013. The Codex Alimentarius for gluten adopted by the European Union is also 20 ppm, and Canada uses the same standard.

What Is Cross-Contamination and Why Should I Care?

It would be wonderful if we could see gluten in food, if it was a certain shade of green or purple or had a specific shape all its own, or if we could perform simple home testing. Unfortunately, we can't. We have to become gluten-free savvy so we know how to avoid it in its various forms. Labels on our products and protocols set up in restaurants go a long way to help us stay safe, but we still need to know how to spot dietary pitfalls.

One of the biggest unknowns for folks on a GFD is not the food itself but cross-contamination. Anytime gluten-free food comes in contact with gluten, you run the risk of cross-contamination, which can be as detrimental to your health as intentionally eating gluten. Crumbs of gluten can linger on shared equipment, such as toasters, grills, fryers, cooking surfaces, preparation countertops, cooling racks, and utensils. Shared condiment jars, peanut butter jars, cheese spreads, and butter sticks or tubs can harbor the remains of gluteny foods just waiting to latch onto a clean knife and land on your gluten-free bread.

One of the worst culprits is the large pot of hot pasta water that sits on the back burner of many restaurant stoves. As the night wears on and more pasta is cooked in this pot, the water gets gummier and cloudier. It's full of gluten that has leached from all that pasta. Then the cook cooks your "gluten-free" pasta or blanches vegetables in that water and puts them on your plate where he or she has carefully placed a gluten-free steak. Those seemingly safe and healthy veggies are now coated with enough gluten to ruin your night. (See "Six Dangerous Places in a Restaurant Kitchen," page 196.)

Gluten-free means not only gluten-free ingredients and products, but also extends to foods prepared free of cross-contamination and also being served and stored away from those that contain gluten. (Gluten-free crackers arranged on the same cheese platter as wheat crackers? That gluten-free cookie next to the "conventional" cookie in the bakery case? Probably not a good idea.)

Bottom line: Getting gluten into your food through cross-contamination can easily make you as sick as eating a piece of bread.

Cross-Contamination Is Real!

A study done by the Center for Celiac Research focused entirely on cross-contamination. The researchers worked with a small group of diagnosed patients with celiac disease who were not recovering despite being on a GFD. They removed all commercially prepared gluten-free foods (i.e., potential for cross-contamination) and put the patients on very plain, simple foods, such as baked chicken and potatoes, for three to six months. Fourteen of the seventeen patients in the study responded to the "Gluten Contamination Elimination Diet" and eleven of those individuals were able to return to a traditional gluten-free diet without the return of symptoms or elevated blood levels, according to the report.[3]

Raising Your GF IQ:
Foods That Are Usually Safe but Sound Scary

Corn and rice gluten

These two are tricky. Corn and rice both contain gluten, but the structure is totally different and not a kind that will trigger a reaction in people with celiac disease or gluten sensitivity. Nevertheless, people often freak out when they see "corn gluten" listed on an ingredient list or buy short-grain rice only to notice its label says "glutinous rice" in parentheses. It's okay. You can have these.

Oats

For years, oats were lumped with wheat, rye, and barley and we were told they were unsafe for a GFD. Then food scientists determined that the amino acid chain is different and that the reason oats were not safe is that farmers rotate their oat crop with wheat and use the same harvesting and storing facilities. Despite the fact that oats could most likely be digested by people with celiac disease, testing of the commercial products found significant amounts of gluten. Today, several companies in North America (see page 313) produce gluten-free oats. These are grown in dedicated fields and harvested and processed on dedicated machinery They are safe for most people who are celiac or gluten sensitive and the federal regulations permit oats containing less than 20 ppm of gluten to be labeled "gluten-free." Celiac patients should consult their physicians before using oats, as some people have issues with the high amount of fiber.

Wheat starch

Wheat starch is washed to remove the gluten. However, despite the processing, some gluten remains. In some parts of Europe, "gluten-free" wheat starch is used in products and the Codex Alimentarius allows it to be labeled "very low-gluten," meaning the product may contain between 21 and 100 ppm of gluten; or labeled "gluten-free," meaning the product tests below 20 ppm. We do not have a low-gluten standard in the United States. However, if wheat starch is used in a product in the United States and the product tests below 20 ppm, it can be labeled "gluten-free" even if the wheat starch, alone, would not test below 20 ppm. People with a wheat allergy may still have problems with products containing this amount of wheat starch.

Caramel coloring and caramel flavoring

In the United States, caramel color and flavor are derived from corn. Occasionally caramel in imported products is made from barley, but that rarely happens as manufacturers prefer corn. You'll see caramel color and flavor listed in a lot of food products.

Annatto

Annatto is used both as a spice and as a natural food coloring. Sometimes it is used as a color in caramel coloring. But, no worries—it is gluten-free.

Vinegar

Vinegar is in everything from ketchup to pickles, cocktail sauce, and relish. Years ago, anyone with celiac was told to avoid "white" vinegar as it was made using grain alcohol. We now know that the gluten molecule is too large to pass through the distillation filters when the vinegar is processed. That means it's safe for people on a gluten-free diet. Many condiments and salad dressings that were off the table have been returned to us, thanks to this revelation. The only exception is malt vinegar, which is fermented with barley and not distilled and is on the list of foods to avoid. Additionally, many of the major manufacturers (e.g., Heinz) have always used white vinegar that's made from corn alcohol.

Watch out for flavored vinegar, however, as it might contain additional ingredients. Most balsamic vinegar is made from grape must and juice, so it is perfectly safe. However, I have seen one balsamic vinegar, a domestic restaurant product, which contains wheat. Stick to the imported brands and be sure to double-check labels.

Blue cheese

It's usually okay. Blue cheese was traditionally made by injecting bread mold into the cheese to create the blue veins; hence, blue cheese. Today, the mold spores are manufactured in a lab. No bread is involved. A few artisan cheeses still use the traditional bread mold and declare "contains wheat" on the package. Gorgonzola, Roquefort, and Stilton also fall into this category. (Recent testing by Health Canada showed no detectable gluten in any brands.)

Adhesive on envelopes and stamps

This rumor keeps circulating like an undeliverable postcard. Every time it rears its ugly head, I return to my sources to see whether something has changed. But, no. Licking envelopes and stamps is safe. According to the Envelope Manufacturers Association, envelope glue does not contain gluten. In fact there are only a few envelope glue makers in the United States and the largest one makes its adhesive from corn. More than 98 percent of all stamps sold by the US Postal Service are self-adhesive and do not require licking. The other 2 percent do not contain gluten in the glue.

Grain-fed poultry and meat

Don't worry; you don't have to become vegetarian, too. In this case, you are not what you eat. The feed that's given to animals goes through their digestive tract, where the nutrients are absorbed into the blood and transported to other parts of the animal's body very much the way it's done in the human system. We eat the muscle from the animal. Gluten itself is not absorbed into the bloodstream. So, no need to put down your knife and fork. Being gluten-free does not mean giving up meat.

Rice (does it contain arsenic?)

For months, make that years, we've heard that the level of arsenic in rice *might* pose a health risk. It's been especially worrisome for people on a gluten-free diet. After all, everything we eat seems to be rice-based.

But the FDA recently tested more than 1,300 samples of rice and rice products and found that, although the levels of arsenic vary, overall, they are too low to cause any immediate or short-term harm. The highest levels are in brown rice (160 parts per billion), which is no surprise, as most of the arsenic accumulates in the hull of the rice kernel.

Arsenic occurs naturally in the soil worldwide. Most crops don't absorb it, but rice that grows in flooded fields is known for taking up large amounts of arsenic. The amount varies by local conditions. California rice has lower arsenic levels than does rice from Texas and Arkansas.

The FDA has not established safe levels for arsenic in rice. The agency is conducting a risk assessment to consider how much rice and rice products Americans eat and whether there is any risk due to long-term exposure.

Meanwhile, the operative word is *diversify*. Eat rice and don't worry. But switch it up by incorporating other gluten-free grains, such as quinoa, buckwheat, and amaranth), into your diet.

Food Myths That Could Make You Sick

It's okay to eat the cheese off regular pizza.

Please, don't do that. Pulling the cheese off pizza and lapping the frosting off birthday cakes would be considered cross-contamination of the highest magnitude. When that gluten-filled pizza bakes and the cheese melts and drapes across the surface, or when it is being cut with the gluten-contaminated cutting wheel, it is collecting gluten molecules. If you pull off the cheese layer, you are devouring a layer of gluten, too. So, don't fall for it as I did. (Yes, in my early days on the GFD, I ate the cheese off pizza.) Many places offer yummy gluten-free pizza (safe from cross-contamination) and gluten-free birthday cake. So treat yourself and avoid gluten exposure.

A chef told me semolina is okay.

Semolina and durum are both forms of wheat. These are full of gluten. But some well-meaning people think a product label has to state "wheat" to be included on the list of no's. It's like convincing them that all-purpose flour and whole wheat flour are *both* from wheat; or their trying to tell you that because something is made from "whole-grain flour," it's good for you. No matter how you slice it, it's still gluten.

Farro is gluten-free.

Farro, an ancient grain, is not gluten-free, but it is much lower in gluten than wheat. Some chefs confuse low gluten with no gluten and mistakenly try to insist that farro is gluten-free. People with mild gluten sensitivity or wheat allergy might be able to tolerate farro. Check with your physician, first. Gluten avoiders may decide to enjoy this nutritious grain or not.

Couscous or fregula is okay; they're not a grain.

Fregula is Sardinian pasta—very similar to Israeli couscous. It and couscous (the larger Israeli and the smaller Italian forms) are full of wheat. This option is *not* available to those with wheat allergy or gluten sensitivity, either. Gluten avoiders should also avoid fregula and couscous if they are avoiding all wheat products.

Freekeh is gluten-free.

An ancient form of wheat that's making a comeback, freekeh is young, green wheat that's been toasted and cracked and makes great grain-filled dishes. But, unfortunately, it's not gluten-free.

Spelt is safe for people with celiac disease.

Spelt is another form of ancient wheat. It's lower in gluten and might be tolerated by people with a wheat allergy. It is not safe for people with celiac disease or gluten sensitivity, but well-meaning natural food store clerks are forever foisting spelt bagels and pretzels on us, saying they are gluten-free.

Sprouted wheat is gluten-free.

Sprouted or germinated wheat still has the protein present. It is not safe.

Kamut is gluten-free.

Like spelt and farro, this is another form of wheat. It is lower in gluten and may be tolerated by those with wheat allergies, but people with celiac disease must stay clear. If you are gluten sensitive and can sometimes tolerate small amounts of gluten, try these forms first. Gluten avoiders may want to partake of this nutritious grain or not.

Note: Under FALCPA, if a product contains farro, freekeh, fregula, kamut, semolina, or spelt, it must say "contains wheat" on the product label.

Heating foods removes the gluten.

This myth seems to be rampant in the restaurant world, but it is just plain bunk. Heat does not remove gluten.

When bread rises, the gluten evaporates.

Actually, it is the elasticity in the gluten that helps the bread rise. This one is not true. If it was, why would we need gluten-free bread?

This is vegan. You'll be fine.

It's not meat—it's wheat! Many restaurants lump all the special diets into one and offer a separate, vegan menu with a few gluten-free items. This could be another opportunity for miscommunication. Best to cross-examine your server to be sure he or she understands your diet. Sometimes people will say their food is "all natural" or "glucose-free," so it's safe. Nice sentiment, but what does that have to do with gluten?

Wheatgrass and barley grass are safe for a GFD.

The grasses are technically gluten-free. These are the young form of the plant, before they mature and turn into the grain or seed where the protein lives. Many manufacturers claim there is no gluten in wheat- and barley grass. Because these grasses hang out with wheat, who's to say if there isn't some cross-contamination going on among the grasses and the grains, given the fact that not every plant matures at the same time. Just avoid them.

Note: Tricia Thompson, MS, RD, has a website discussion on this topic at glutenfreedietician.com.

Gluten, Gluten Everywhere

I'm fond of saying, "I can eat from the major food groups: wine, coffee, chocolate, and potato chips!" But as you have a sense by now, there are a lot of groups—food and otherwise—that aren't so safe for us. Here's the lowdown on booze, medication, and personal care products.

Alcoholic Beverages

Gluten in Grain-Based Spirits

You've been told you need to be on a GFD and the worst thing is that you have to give up those martinis and single malt Scotch. Well, don't toss the shaker just yet. That martini and the single malt scotch are safe for your diet. It turns out that distilled alcohol does not contain gluten, because the gluten molecules are too large to pass through the filter in the distillation process. There are a few exceptions. (Don't you wish everything about this diet was black and white?)

You'll still need to avoid liquors that add back a bit of mash (from grain) for color and flavor. The process is done *after* distillation. In addition, some alcohol is infused with flavors that are not gluten-free. Check with the manufacturer about its process if there is any doubt. Generally, the less expensive brands are more suspect.

Most liqueurs are gluten-free, including brandy, cognac, port, sherry, and grappa (all made from grapes). Although technically these are not spirits, you can add hard cider and gluten-free beers to that list as well.

Avoid blended liqueurs, some cordials, and some wine coolers (which may contain malt) as these are not gluten-free. Again, check with each manufacturer on this last group.

Why Do Some People Think That Grain Alcohol Is Unsafe?

Perhaps alcohol gets a bad rap because the distillation process is not monitored, so there's no way to say for certain that100 percent of the gluten is removed. Still, most of the leading organizations say that all distilled alcohol is gluten-free regardless of the grains used, as no gluten protein remains after it's distilled. That position is shared by the Canadian Celiac Association, the National Institutes of Health Celiac Disease Awareness Campaign, and several patient support groups. The Academy of Nutrition and Dietetics (formerly the American Dietetic Association) also supports this position.

Still worried about taking a nip of something that started out as a gluten-containing grain? Try one of the alcoholic beverages made from gluten-free grains, such as vodka made from potatoes, rum, tequila (from corn and cactus), wines, brandies, and gluten-free beers.

My take? Well, I love wine and rarely drink hard liquor. I am not sure if that stems back to decades ago when we thought grain alcohol contained gluten or because I love wine and there are so many vineyards making wonderful products. But I understand your passion if your drink of choice has always been Scotch or bourbon. You'll just have to be mindful when you drink (in more ways than one).

Uncorking the Truth: Is There Wheat in Wine?

Of course, wine, itself, is naturally gluten-free. It's just grapes, after all, so it's the go-to drink for many of us. But it's the process that raises some worries among gluten-free folks who enjoy a glass of vino.

Traditionally, wineries used oak barrels in making most wines, especially the reds that need to age the longest. Vintners are moving away from oak barrels because of cost, maintenance, and availability. Many white wines and some younger reds are aged in stainless steel. But cabernet sauvignon, merlot, and zinfandel can still be aged in oak barrels, and these are sometimes sealed with wheat paste. Does that contaminate the wine? Well, most likely, no. Even wine that is aged in oak barrels is not really at risk, as only the barrel heads are sealed with paste and the amount used is tiny, so there's limited exposure of wheat to wine. Besides, all barrels are pressure-washed with boiling water before they are used, removing any residual paste.

So, How Much Gluten Gets into Wine?

Tricia Thompson, MS, RD (The Gluten-free Dietitian, glutenfreedietitian .com), tested two wines, a cabernet sauvignon and a merlot, which were aged in wheat-sealed oak barrels at the same vineyard. She used two very sensitive types of testing (Competitive R5 ELISA and Sandwich R5 ELISA), and the wines tested to below 10 and below 5 parts per million of gluten, respectively.

What's Brewing with Beer

Beer is a subject that is much less clear cut. Beer is fermented (not distilled) and traditionally made with barley hops. (Okay, some of it's made from wheat or rye, too.) The gluten in barley, called hordein, is a no-no if you are seriously gluten-free (celiac or gluten sensitive).

Because beer has never been considered safe for people on a gluten-free diet, more than a dozen companies produce designer, gluten-free beers. These are started with gluten-free grains, such as sorghum, millet, rice, and corn, and they are all safe for people on a gluten-free diet. They never contained gluten.

But the taste of these alternative grains has never quite satisfied true beer connoisseurs. And now, several beer companies throughout the world are producing gluten-reduced barley-based beer. Omission Beer from Oregon, Two Brothers Prairie Path Golden Ale from Illinois, and Estrella Damm Daura from Spain use a proprietary brewing method that can *de-gluten* barley beer and bring the gluten level down well below 20 ppm, using the R5 ELISA test results. Tasters claim it tastes like real beer.

An enzyme that has been used by craft brewers around the world as a clarifying agent works to break down proteins, including gluten, in the beer.[1] But it's not adding clarity to the issue about whether barley-based gluten-free beers are actually safe.

Concerns About Barley-Based Beer

Gluten is a complex protein, made up of smaller proteins, including gliadin, hordein, and glutelin. The protein is broken down into its smaller components. But there is some question about whether the gluten is actually removed. It's not detectable in the laboratory tests, but is it detectable in the body?

Dr. Steve L. Taylor, cofounder and director of the Food Allergy Research and Resource Program (FARRP), believes that barley-based beers might contain peptides (large fragments) of gluten that could possibly still be hazardous to people with celiac disease. "The results from the R5 test alone do not convince me that they are safe. I have seen results that show the gluten peptides do exist in these beers."

Several barley-based beers were tested, using the mass spectrometry method, and the results were published in the *Journal of Proteome Research*, from the American Chemical Society.[2]

In the study, scientists used mass spectrometry to examine hordein protein levels in sixty different beers, including some that were labeled "gluten-free barley beer." This method is expensive and not widely used. But it seems to be more reliable for determining whether the hordein remains in barley-containing beers.

The results: beers labeled "low-gluten" (not identified by brand) did not necessarily have less gluten than some nonlabeled beers.[3]

Recent tests by Health Canada had similar findings. They "found gluten fragments in beers from Spain and Belgium that use a gluten-removal process similar to Craft Brew's [Omission Beer]," reports an article in the

Oregonian, June 8, 2013. "It's unclear whether the fragments are a health concern," says a Health Canada spokesperson in the article.[4]

I think Dr. Taylor summed it up when he said, "Uncertainty and a lack of suitable analytical methods surround this subject, so I just think people with celiac disease should drink barley-based beer with caution."[5]

Who Regulates Gluten-free Beer?

The Alcohol, Tobacco Tax and Trade Bureau (TTB) that regulates beer and distilled alcoholic beverages permits gluten-free labeling claims only on products made from gluten-free ingredients, such as vodka distilled only from potatoes. In an interim policy issued in May 2012 and recon-firmed after the FDA released its gluten-free labeling rule, TTB will not allow de-gluten-ed beers to be labeled "gluten-free." It does allow the fol-lowing statement: "crafted to remove gluten." However, the label must also state that the product was fermented (or distilled) from grains con-taining gluten. The label must also carry a warning that says "no test exists to verify gluten in beer."[6]

Look to the FDA which has jurisdiction over gluten-free labeling rules for food, to address the issue of fermented or hydrolyzed products includ-ing beers in a future ruling.

Gluten and Medication

Things to Know About Medications, Over-the-Counter (OTC) Medicines, Vitamins, and Other Dietary Supplements

Is there gluten in your prescription meds, cough syrup, or vitamins? Is it okay to drink the barium mixture for an upper GI X-ray? What about the elixirs used for a colonoscopy prep or the mouthwash recommended by the dentist?

These are gray areas, indeed, and not covered by FALCPA, the FDA gluten-free labeling regulations, or the Food, Drug and Cosmetic Act. What follows is the good and bad news about medications and how to sort through the drug labyrinth. Dietary supplements and vitamins that carry the gluten-free label fall under the FDA gluten-free labeling rule. While companies are not required to state "gluten-free" on their products, if they do, you will know they are safe. If they don't, well, you'll need to dig further. Much of the following information will be helpful in your detective work.

Gut Reaction: Can That Tiny Pill Really Hurt Me?

Not only do I have celiac disease, but I also have hypothyroidism. It's not unusual.

Here's the deal. The medication most often prescribed to treat this is either Levoxyl or Synthroid. Mine is Synthroid. It's stabilized my thyroid stimulating hormone (TSH) levels and my celiac antibodies are always normal. Okay. That should be the end of this discussion. But it's only the beginning. When I visit DailyMed, the NIH website that lists all medications and most of the sources of the inactive ingredients, there's nothing questionable in the ingredient list.

The original manufacturer of Synthroid, Flint, said the medication was gluten-free. While the formula has not changed, the new owner, Abbott, chooses not to make that statement since it doesn't do final testing. On the other hand, King Pharmaceuticals, the makers of Levoxyl, says its product is gluten-free.

So why not simply switch to the one I know is safe? Well, thyroid medications are not easily interchangeable. The therapeutic window is very narrow. Varying the time of day the pill is taken or switching brands of medication can affect the dose. Switching might mean I'd have to start all over again trying to regulate my thyroid function.

My physician doesn't want me to switch medications, either: "Really, how much gluten could possibly be in that tiny pill even if there was some gluten in one of the ingredients?" she says. She has a point.

I still wasn't sold; then I noticed that someone on the Celiac Listserv asked the same question. The reply from Steven Plogsted, Pharm-D, caught my attention. Dr. Plogsted, an expert on gluten in medications, is a doctor of pharmacy and a clinical pharmacist at Nationwide Children's Hospital in Columbus, Ohio. He also created glutenfreedrugs.com, an essential website for anyone who needs a

▶

gluten-free diet and takes medication. He was saying the same thing my physician had told me.

"First, if there is a starch, there is only a slight possibility it is derived from wheat. If it is, the amount is probably not measurable," said Dr. Plogsted when I spoke to him. He points to the Catassi and Fasano study that established the 50 mg of gluten or 20 ppm threshold of gluten as being safe for most celiac patients.[7]

"The size of your entire tablet probably weighs less than that," says Dr. Plogsted.

It eased my mind. Nevertheless, if anything ever goes wrong gluten-wise, Synthroid will be on my list of suspects.

Gluten Labeling in Medications

The Food, Drug and Cosmetic Act requires that OTC medications list all inactive ingredients in the drug on the "Drug Facts" panel on the medication's container. Prescription drugs, too, must include a list of the inactive ingredients in the package insert. So, it stands to reason that we should be able to read the label and tell whether the drug contains gluten. But there are no regulations requiring drug manufacturers to list the source of inactive ingredients (also called excipients). Neither FALCPA nor the FDA gluten-free labeling rule covers OTC or prescription medications. (The FDA rule does include dietary supplements.)

What we do know is that only about 30 percent of all medications truly contain any starch to begin with. That doesn't mean you are off the hook, however. With more than 150,000 prescription medications in use, according to a paper by Dr. Walter Modell of Cornell University, in *Clinical Pharmacology and Therapeutics*, a substantial number still contain starch. The starches are mainly derived from corn, followed by potato, then tapioca, and lastly, wheat, says Dr. Plogsted.

Other ingredients to watch for include maltodextrin and dextrins. There's a chance they could contain a tiny amount of wheat if they come from another country. And it's possible that mannitol and sorbitol could be derived from wheat, but once the ingredient is manufactured, no protein remains; so, no gluten. They are safe.

Clear liquid medications and gel-caps are made from the sugar in the starch. There's no protein and therefore no gluten here. Rarely is the source of sugars or sugar alcohols a problem. Check with the manufacturer when in doubt.

Still, some drug companies are adopting the disclaimer language, although there is little chance there is gluten in medications, says Dr. Plogsted. "But we are getting less than full disclosure from the drug companies," he says.

Be a detective. While the information here is meant to give you some peace of mind, you may still need to play detective before taking medicine, as a small percentage of medications do contain a form of gluten. That small amount, taken every day for an extended period of time, can add a gluten load to your diet, compounded if something else with gluten is getting into your diet at the same time. So investigate further if the source of inactive ingredients is questionable. And you'll need to be cautious if your medication is a generic brand. The information that comes next will help you sort this out.

Sources of Inactive Ingredients

When the source of the inactive ingredient is not identified, it's important to investigate further. There may be other drugs available from other sources that certify they are gluten-free.

Ask your pharmacist to help you find an equivalent medication from another manufacturer or opt for a liquid version of the medication, if available. These rarely contain gluten. Here's some help in sorting through the sources of inactive ingredients.

Usually safe:

- Cornstarch
- Dextrin (source not specified, but usually from corn or potato)
- Sodium starch glycolate (derived from potato or corn)

Unknown—more information is required:

- Caramel coloring (source could be barley malt if produced in another country)
- Dextrates (unspecified)
- Dextrimaltose (source could be barley malt)
- Maltodextrin and dextrins (there's a slight chance these can be from wheat, especially if the ingredient is produced in another country)
- Modified starch (unspecified)
- Pregelatinized modified starch (unspecified)
- Pregelatinized starch (unspecified)
- Starch (could be wheat)

Note: Part of this list came from information at celiaccentral.org. Also, Dr. Plogsted says he has never seen barley or rye used in drugs.

Changing Formulas

If a company lists "starch," rather than specifying the source (e.g., cornstarch), it can change suppliers as long as the same dose of the medication is delivered each time and through each medium. If it specifies the kind of starch, the company is required to resubmit paperwork and testing to the FDA before it can obtain approval to switch to another specific ingredient.

Generic Drugs

The generic version of a medication can be just as effective as the brand name drug; and sometimes one is gluten-free, while the other is unwilling to make that claim. In fact, some manufacturers also produce the generic brand and sell it to another company. The off-label company that distributes the generic medication might test for gluten in the product, whereas the manufacturer of the labeled product does not.

Don't assume that the generic form is made the same way with the same inactive ingredients. What's more, the generic form can come from more than one supplier and use more than one set of ingredients. It can change each time you fill the prescription. You may need to put on your detective hat each time you pick up the prescription.

Generic medications are typically cheaper, so your insurance company prefers you use them. In fact, some insist on it.

The policy on generic versus brand name drugs varies from state to state. Do your homework before you need your medication. Most likely, you will need to call your insurance carrier or check its website.

The physician can help by writing one of these statements on the prescription:

- Patient has celiac disease
- No substitution
- "DAW" (dispense as written)
- Do not fill with generic brand

Sometimes that is all it takes. For some of the more expensive medications, you might have to appeal up the chain of decision-makers in your insurance company. Don't give up and save all the documentation. This might be a battle you need to wage again.

Tip: Do the research ahead of time. Ask to see the insert and make your calls or check websites *before* buying the prescription. Once the prescription has been picked up, even if it's never used, you can't return it.

Don't be tempted to use online pharmacies to purchase your medication. You have no way of knowing how the medication was made, what fillers were used, and whether you are actually receiving the medication you ordered.

Cross-Contamination

While this is a big issue in food manufacturing, it should not be a concern when it comes to drug manufacturing. Although some drug companies may claim they cannot guarantee there is no cross-contamination in a medication, drug manufacturing is done in sterile rooms, following stringent Food and Drug Administration (FDA) requirements. The companies use stainless steel and the most popular drugs are manufactured alone in dedicated rooms. If two drugs are manufactured in the same room, the FDA protocol requires careful clean-down procedures. These regulations are aiming at more important issues than gluten. If grains of an antipsychotic medication happen to get into a production of antibiotics, the potential health risk to the American public would be amazing.

Not All Digestive Issues Are Celiac

Some medications, particularly antibiotics, can cause upset stomach and diarrhea. It's easy to confuse these with celiac symptoms and believe your medication contains gluten. Check the package insert that comes with your prescription to find out what side effects are likely to occur while taking the medication. Some, such as antibiotics, warn that they can cause digestive symptoms.

Benicar (olmesartan), a blood pressure medication taken by millions, was recently reported to cause celiac-like symptoms (chronic diarrhea and weight loss) in some people. The symptom crossover has led physicians to mistakenly diagnose celiac disease and recommend a GFD and caused some celiac patients to search frantically for hidden sources of gluten in their diet. The drug now carries a warning, and the good news is that most symptoms reversed when people were taken off Benicar.

Other Places to Watch Out for Gluten

- Barium swallow. Some are safe and others are not. Ask the radiology technician to order a safe brand for you well ahead of the date of your procedure. Ask to read the manufacturer's insert prior to downing the drink, to be sure it's the correct product and that it's safe for your diet.
- Elixirs for colonoscopy prep. Every doctor has his or her preferred products. Check all ingredients before you begin the prep. There are likely alternative products that are safe and just as effective.
- Dentist office visits. Some polishing pastes, fluoride treatments, and even mouthwash might contain gluten. Ask the dentist to order safe products well ahead of your visit.

Avoiding Medication Mix-ups

Make sure that medications prescribed by the pharmacist, the physician, or a technician administering a procedure are the correct ones for you. Mix-ups happen all the time. Even if there is a note in your computerized file that you require a GFD, it might go unnoticed. Be vigilant and double-check.

Speaking of computers, if your physician's practice has a patient portal that you can access on your own computer, check to see whether your gluten-related condition and restrictions are listed correctly. After you and your doctor have researched and determined the safe medications for you, the doctor can write specific instructions so there will be no mix-ups at the pharmacy. Remind the doctor each time you visit, to ensure you receive proper medications.

Add the pharmacist to your team of watchdogs who can help you stay clear of risky ingredients in medications. Be sure your gluten-related condition is on file with your pharmacist if the pharmacy has that capability. Most pharmacists are very helpful in researching inactive ingredients for you.

Changing the Dose

If you are on a medication before being diagnosed with celiac disease, you may need to have the dose adjusted once your gut heals and your absorption improves. That's particularly true for medications with a narrow therapeutic range, such as blood thinners, and antiseizure, thyroid, and diabetes medications.

Over-the-Counter (OTC) Drugs

The FDA does not require companies to test products for gluten in OTC drugs. Your best bet is to read the inactive ingredient list and call the company or check its website to determine whether the product is safe.

The good news is that some manufacturers are voluntarily testing and labeling their OTC medications. McNeil (Tylenol) and Perrigo (maker of products for CVS, Walgreens, and other drugstore chains), have both made this commitment.

Walgreens has compiled a list of all its gluten-free OTC medications. Check with the pharmacist on duty or visit the website. CVS Pharmacy also has an extensive list of gluten-free private-label items. For information, go to the CVS website and type in the six-digit code above the UPC code of a product or call the customer service number for assistance.

Vitamins and Supplements

Dietary supplements fall under FALCPA and are also covered by the new voluntary FDA gluten-free labeling regulations. Many manufacturers of vitamins and supplements voluntarily state that their products are gluten-free. If they do not call out this claim, it doesn't mean the product is not gluten-free. In addition, often a supplement is offered by more than one manufacturer and at least one lists "gluten-free" on the label.

Who Needs Vitamins?

If you have celiac disease, you may be deficient in many vitamins and nutrients, especially at first. As the gut heals, some of those levels will return to normal but you may still need to add supplements to maintain optimum health. A survey conducted by a group of German researchers found that people with celiac disease are low on six specific vitamins and minerals: B_1 (thiamine), B_2 (riboflavin), B_6, folic acid, magnesium, and iron.

Although the research was conducted on celiac patients who may always have some diminished capacity to absorb vitamins and nutrients, this would be true for anyone who is not eating gluten-containing products, such as bread and cereal that are often fortified with these vitamins and minerals.

The study recommends regular monitoring to check these levels, so add this to your checklist of health related issues to discuss with your health-care provider.

Picking Good Vitamins

Christine Doherty, ND, a celiac patient, and health practitioner who specializes in celiac disease and gluten sensitivity, adds vitamin D to the list of important vitamins and suggests taking a B-complex supplement as well as magnesium. Because not all supplements are created equal, Doherty has some tips for selecting good quality vitamins. Avoid supplements that contain a superlong list of ingredients that are hard to read and pronounce, she says. Look for vitamin D_3 (cholecalciferol) instead of synthetic D_2 (ergocalciferol); and if you take vitamin E, choose the natural d-alpha-tocopherol form, not the synthetic dl-alpha-tocopherol form.

At a minimum, take a high-quality multivitamin, ideally one that is taken more than once a day, because you will absorb more if you divide the doses with meals, she says. Minerals, such as calcium, are very bulky, so it is impossible to fit a therapeutic dose of even one of them into a one-a-day pill. Most once daily vitamins are low in minerals for this reason.

Doherty recommends taking calcium supplements that include magnesium and even vitamin K, all of which are in many bone support formulas. Purchase a chelated form of the mineral, calcium citrate (as opposed to carbonate), which can be better absorbed. Calcium can be very constipating, and magnesium can be a laxative, so if you have ongoing digestive sensitivity, you may need to adjust your levels for ideal bowel tolerance, she advises.

It's important to know the doses in your B-complex vitamins, especially when taking them in addition to a multivitamin, she warns. If you are taking multiple supplements, it is wise to take an inventory of how much of certain nutrients you are getting, because there is often repetition, and before you know it you can be getting too much or certain nutrients, such as selenium, zinc, niacin, or vitamin B_6, which can then cause such symptoms as digestive upset (selenium, zinc), rashes (niacin), or tingling in your hands and feet (B_6).

For a list of companies that manufacture gluten-free dietary supplements, go to Resources (page 314).

Up the Nose/Through the Skin

Medications, such as lotions, which are absorbed through the skin are not problematic for people with celiac disease, DH, or gluten sensitivity.

If you have a wheat allergy, however, watch out for topical medications that contain these ingredients.

Inhalers and nose drops do not contain wheat and gluten. But the presence of one of the sugar alcohols causes some manufacturers to think these contain gluten when, in fact, they are safe, says Dr. Plogsted.

What Are Sugar Alcohols?

Sugar alcohols are not truly sugars or alcohols. They are naturally found in a number of fruits and vegetables and may be extracted from many sources, including wheat. During the manufacturing process, they are completely refined, leaving behind no gluten proteins. Sugar alcohols include mannitol and xylitol, which are both considered gluten-free.

Helpful Resources

Knowing what to ask and who to ask, gets you past the gatekeepers.

—Dr. Steven Plogsted

Daily Med. Published by National Institutes of Health (NIH), this is a service of the federal government. It is updated on a regular basis and discloses the source of inactive ingredients for many drugs. DailyMed.nlm.nih.gov.

The Physician's Desk Reference (PDR). The PDR lists every prescription medication made as well as the ingredients, active and inactive. It won't tell you the source of starches in your particular prescription. But it includes a customer service toll-free number for each product. The customer service person might not know the sources of starches, but you can ask to speak with the research chemist associated with that drug. The PDR is a huge book and expensive, too. Use its online service (drugs.com/pdr) or borrow the PDR from the pharmacist where you fill your medications. Most of the information in the PDR is also in the product insert that should come with your medication.

Gluten-free Drugs. Glutenfreedrugs.com is a website that lists of gluten-free drugs maintained by Dr. Steven Plogsted and his pharmacy students at Nationwide Children's Hospital in Columbus, Ohio. It's a vital research tool for those of us who are gluten-free.

National Foundation for Celiac Awareness. CeliacCentral.org, the website of the National Foundation for Celiac Awareness (NFCA), has a section devoted to gluten in medications and works closely with the American Pharmacists Association (APhA).

Gluten in Medications Guide. This guide is available at celiaccentral.org and maintained by the NFCA. It was created in collaboration with the American Society of Health-System Pharmacists (ASHP) and provides helpful tips for what to ask pharmacists about gluten-free prescriptions and other medication needs.

Watch for future legislation: The Gluten in Medication Disclosure Act was introduced in Congress by Congressman Tim Ryan (D-OH) and Congresswoman Nita Lowey (D-NY). If passed, this legislation will require drug companies to identify the source of starch in their drugs.

The Skinny on Cosmetics:
Skin Care Products and Lipstick

Even people with DH do not need to avoid skin care products, only products that go on the lips and might be swallowed.

—STEFANO GUANDALINI, MD, FOUNDER AND MEDICAL DIRECTOR,
CELIAC DISEASE CENTER, UNIVERSITY OF CHICAGO

At an American College of Gastroenterology meeting in early 2013, researchers reported, "No evidence that gluten in skin care products is harmful to people with celiac disease or gluten sensitivity. That's true even for those who tend to develop skin rashes when exposed to gluten in foods. Unless you have sores on your skin, it's unlikely that much gluten from lotion or makeup would enter your system."[8]

Okay. Why are we having this discussion, anyway? Well, gluten in lotions and cosmetics is a hot button for seriously gluten-free folks. Many believe that gluten-containing lotions and cosmetics are harmful, despite the evidence to the contrary.

So, do you need to avoid them or not? Mostly, no. Lotions and creams are absorbed through the skin and not through the mouth (the gatekeeper to the digestive system). Unless you are licking your skin, which sounds kind of kinky anyway, you don't need to worry. Even if you want to get kinky, most of this stuff has been absorbed after a couple of hours. We'll talk about licking someone else's skin in Chapter 13.

Lipstick and Lip Gloss

The exception is if products can get into your mouth (i.e., lip care products). Even then, some studies show there is not enough gluten in lip care items to trigger a reaction. (A study in the *Journal of the Academy of Nutrition and Dietetics* reported that a range of lip products had tested well below the 20 ppm of gluten.)

But the notion of smearing wheat germ oil all over my lips is still unnerving. If you are like me, you'll want the latest information—the skinny on lotions, skin creams, and cosmetics—so you can make educated decisions.

What Form of Gluten Is Found in Skin Creams, Lotions, and Cosmetics?

Here are a few ingredients derived from gluten. (The ingredients are listed on the container or on the outside packaging.) As mentioned earlier, these ingredients are generally recognized as safe in topical products for anyone with CD, DH, or GS; however, some people prefer to take no chances and avoid these gluteny ingredients altogether. Anyone with a wheat allergy should avoid the ingredients derived from wheat.

- Avena sativa (oats)
- Barley
- Barley extract
- *Hordeum vulgare* (barley)
- Malt

- Oats
- Oat kernel flour
- Rye
- *Secale cereale* (rye)
- Tocopherol (can be from wheat)
- *Triticum vulgare* (wheat germ oil)
- Vitamin E (can be from wheat)
- Wheat
- Wheat bran extract
- Wheat germ oil
- Wheat germ extract

Hair Products

Unless you sing in the shower, hair products should be safe. Just like skin care products, these cannot be absorbed through the scalp. But you do stand a chance of getting a mouthful of soap when you are rinsing. This is one time that keeping your mouth shut is a good idea.

Facials and Masks

By all means, treat yourself to a facial. However, ask the aesthetician to avoid your mouth. Keep moist tissues handy to wipe away any stray materials from around the lips and mouth area. Alternatively, select only products that do not contain gluten. Or select other spa treatments that don't involve the face. Massage, anyone?

Bottom Line

Many cosmetic and skin care brands now have a list of their gluten-free products. For peace of mind, whenever possible, these are still a safer choice. And if you use products that contain gluten, be sure to wash your hands after applying them.

If you are avoiding gluten by choice, do you need to be mindful of gluten in cosmetics and skin care products? Probably not. But many gluten-free cosmetics are also perfume- and chemical-free, making these a fine choice for anyone. And you'll want to avoid *eating* gluten-containing shampoos, lip products, and facial masks, but you would do that anyway.

Wheat allergic folks *will* need to avoid skin care products that contain wheat, wheat germ oil, and other wheat-derived ingredients (see list on pags 113–114), as these can set off rashes, hives, itching, even sneezing.

Children and Skin Products

Kids put their hands in their mouth and whatever is on those hands goes in, too. Children with gluten or wheat issues should not use skin care products containing gluten. If these products must be used, make sure children wash their hands after applying lotions and creams.

Ready, Set, Shop

You are now armed with a list of ingredients that are safe and those to avoid, the tools to read labels, and how to deal with other circumstances (alcohol, medications, and cosmetics) where gluten can present a problem. Now it's time to shop.

8

❧ Food Shopping

Shopping. You'll do a lot of that now that you're on a GFD. Processed, prepared, and convenience foods are generally not GFF. From a health standpoint, that's a good thing. But you'll probably spend more time shopping and doing more of your own cooking as a result. Don't worry. You can do this.

In "Diet Diligence" (page 82), I listed ingredients that could contain gluten and those that are safe. Thanks to two major changes in the way packaged foods are labeled, one rule of exclusion and the other a rule of inclusion, you don't need a PhD to decipher the world of commercial foods and you no longer need an entire day to study labels and select safe foods.

FALCPA: The Rule of Exclusion

The Food Allergen Labeling and Consumer Protection Act of 2004 (FALCPA) requires food manufacturers to list any of the top eight allergens if they are in a product. Wheat is one of them. This legislation helps to clarify sources of modified food starch, hydrolyzed plant protein, natural flavors, all of which were left for consumers to sort through before the ruling passed. While FALCPA doesn't address gluten per se and doesn't include barley or rye, wheat covers about 90 percent of foods we need to avoid. Unfortunately, it doesn't tell you a product is safe and doesn't address cross-contamination, but it certainly helps in ruling out products. If you see "contains wheat" on the label, put it back. FALCPA only covers FDA-regulated products, which do not include meat, poultry, cold cuts, hot dogs, and some egg products (regulated by the USDA), so read the fine print in those products' ingredient labels extra carefully.

Gluten-free Food Labeling Regulation: The Rule of Inclusion

Required under FALCPA, this takes a big step toward making it easier for gluten-free consumers to shop safely and more efficiently. As of August 2014, companies that wish to make the gluten-free claim on their label must also be able to demonstrate that those products contain less than 20 ppm of gluten. This is a voluntary rule and some companies may choose not to make the gluten-free claim on a product although it is gluten-free. In that case, you still need to check with the company for clarity. Companies can also label foods "gluten-free" that are, by nature, free of gluten (bottled spring water, fresh fruits and vegetables, and fresh seafood). But not all companies label their inherently safe products. That does not mean the others (without a gluten-free claim) are any less safe. (See more on the FDA labeling rule below.)

If a product is labeled "gluten-free," you know it's safe to eat. While this rule makes life easier, you are not entirely off the hook. You will still make your share of calls and search company websites but, believe me, you'll do less detective work than was required in the past.

Things to Know About the FDA Gluten-free Food Labeling Rule

A gluten-free diet for people with celiac disease is like insulin for diabetics.

—ALESSIO FASANO, MD,[1] NEW YORK TIMES, AUGUST 2, 2013

Let's talk about what's covered in this important labeling rule.

- Gluten-containing grains are defined as wheat, rye, barley, and hybrids, such as triticale.

- Oats are considered safe if they are labeled "gluten-free."
- The rule is voluntary. A manufacturer can choose not to call its product "gluten-free" even if it contains no gluten. (If you think a product is safe, but it is not labeled "gluten-free," you might need to call the manufacturer. We'll talk about this again in a moment.)
- Foods labeled "gluten-free" must test below 20 ppm of gluten, the level deemed medically safe for most people with celiac disease.
- Manufacturers are responsible for making sure their products meet all labeling requirements. After August 5, 2014, misbranded food products are subject to regulatory action. Products do not need to follow a specific label format to use the "gluten-free" claim.
- The rule applies to all FDA-regulated foods, including dietary supplements.
- It does not cover food under USDA (meat, poultry, and certain egg products) or products regulated by the TTB (distilled spirits or wines with 7 percent or more alcohol, or malted beverages made with malted barley and hops). However, both the USDA and TTB are working to bring the foods and drinks they regulate in line with the FDA rule.
- The rule does not cover medications.

For more information, go to fda.gov.

Symbol(s) for Gluten-free Foods and What They Mean

Several third-party gluten-free certification programs review manufacturers' products and offer symbols to show that the products meet their standard of gluten-free safety. These provide the "seal of approval" and peace of mind to consumers shopping for gluten-free food. Generally, companies will display only one symbol. The symbol can appear anywhere on the product's package. If a company uses a third-party certification, its label should meet the requirements of the certifying organization as well as the FDA standard of 20 ppm, says the FDA. (For the most popular certification programs, products must test to levels that are lower than the FDA standard.) Here are some of the symbols you might see and what they mean to you.

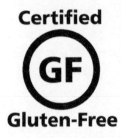

Certified

GF

Gluten-Free

The Gluten-free Certification Organization (GFCO) has certified more than 550 companies and more than 16,600 products. Each product must test below 10 ppm of gluten to use this symbol. Manufacturers go through an initial audit before they are approved. An annual audit is required to assess risk of ingredients and equipment and products are subject to spot review and annual recertification. This program is run by the Gluten Intolerance Group of North America (GIG), www.gluten.net.

The National Foundation for Celiac Awareness (NFCA) has formed an alliance with the GFCP, developed by the Canadian Celiac Association (CCA), to endorse the GFCP in the United States. The program requires gluten-free products to be produced below 10 ppm of gluten. This is verified at the facility as part of a specific GFCP annual management system certification audit,

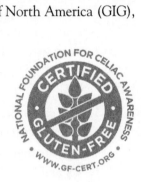

conducted by independent International Organization for Standardization (ISO)–accredited auditing companies. For more information on this NFCA-endorsed program, go to www.gf-cert.org.

Celiac Support Association™

Celiac Support Association, formerly Celiac Sprue Association (CSA) Recognition Program requires foods to have less than 5 ppm of gluten and be free of wheat, rye, barley, and "common" oats. Companies submit the analysis of ingredients and manufacturing procedures to the CSA for review prior to receiving the CSA Recognition Seal. Information on this program is available at www.csaceliacs.info.

Gluten Sensibility

Labeling information is meant to help you. But it's not foolproof. And product labels can change.

Here are three ways to check the gluten-free status of a product:

- Search for information about the company on the Internet. (Type the name of the product and "gluten-free" into the browser.)
- Check the company's gluten-free product list.
- Read the label of the product in question and write down the UPC number that's below the bar code, then call the consumer hotline.

(Un)Truth in Advertising

Don't you wonder who benefits from all those claims made on food packaging? A candy that's full of sugar, food dyes, and artificial flavors calls out "fat-free" as if it's a health food. Or bottled water claims it is "smart" water. Does that imply drinking it will make you smarter?

Some products that look gluten-free might be misleading, too. What does it mean when a product label says "no gluten-containing ingredients," "no gluten," "may contain traces of wheat," or "made in a facility that also manufacturers products containing wheat?" The gluten-free labeling regulation lends some clarity to these and other labeling questions that have been confusing the gluten-free public for years. Take a look at some of the ambiguous issues now clarified.

- "No gluten," "free of gluten," and "without gluten" are synonymous with "gluten-free" when they are used on a product label.
- However, if a product is labeled "made with no gluten-containing ingredients" or "not made with gluten-containing ingredients" but does not say "gluten-free," it is not subject to the FDA rule.
- Products labeled "manufactured in a plant that also processes wheat," but also making the "gluten-free claim," are considered safe.
- Products labeled "manufactured in a plant that also processes wheat," and that do not make the "gluten-free" claim, do not fall under the regulation. They may or may not be safe. Further information is needed.
- Foods with ingredients that are gluten-containing grains that are refined but still contain gluten (e.g., wheat flour) may not be labeled

"gluten-free." Foods (such as wheat starch) that are refined in a way that removes the gluten, may be labeled "gluten-free" as long as the food contains less than 20 ppm gluten.

- Foods can't be labeled "gluten-free" if they contain 20 ppm or more of gluten as a result of cross-contamination.

Gut Reaction: A Monumental Day in DC

It was early spring 2011. The FDA gluten-free labeling rule (mandated by FALCPA legislation) was three years overdue. Celiac patients and gluten-free manufacturers alike were tapping their toes impatiently all over America. The gluten-free frenzy was growing and, with it, products coming to market that called out "gluten-free" and attached a litany of disclaimers. How was a seriously gluten-free person to know what was safe to eat?

Cookbook author and blogger Jules Shepard, web guru John Forberger, professional baker Lee Tobin, head of the Whole Foods Market Gluten-free Bakehouse, and Aaron Flores, executive chef at the Embassy Suites in Washington, DC, decided to build the world's tallest gluten-free cake (more than 11 feet tall—and shaped like the Washington Monument, no less) in the atrium of the hotel. Their tower of confection was aimed at heightening awareness for the growing number of people who have celiac disease (a campaign billed as 1 in 133) and the need for a gluten-free labeling rule to make their food safe.

Jules and company enlisted support from the American Celiac Disease Alliance (ACDA) and invited folks to come to Washington to help frost the cake. Exciting as this event promised to be, frosting a cake was not going to keep everyone busy for the entire day. "Let's harness all that energy. Let's ask congressmen and senators to get the FDA moving on this labeling rule. Let's get the ball rolling," I suggested.

The momentum grew just like the many layers of the monumental cake. Andrea Levario, executive director of the ACDA and our advocate in Washington, set up appointments with congressmen and senators. I corralled gluten-free manufacturers. Everyone called members of the press to tell them our plan. "A march to Capitol Hill [we actually took the Metro] and a giant gluten-free cake party," we tweeted and

▶

blogged. We explained why we needed their help. The energy began to snowball as things will do when there's an important cause, a lot at stake, and nothing to lose. Colleagues were poised and ready to arrive in Washington on May 4, 2011. They had contacted their local congressmen. The cake layers were arriving as was a ton (or so) of frosting. The press took note.

Congressional staffers, senators and representatives had been in touch with the FDA on our behalf. Articles had appeared in media all over the country. The *Washington Post* ran a front-page article on April 28 with a headline that read, "A Gluten-free-For-All: With FDA Rules Overdue, Millions Don't Know Whom to Trust."

As Jules and her team constructed their tower of confection, our delegation (about a dozen people) *swarmed* Capitol Hill. Besides Andrea and me and our sons, there were food manufacturers, such as Glutino, King Arthur Flour, and Nu-World Amaranth, and the executive editor of *Living Without*, Alicia Woodward. Then came the medical and research communities, including the Center for Celiac Research at University of Maryland and the University of Chicago Celiac Disease Center as well as such national support organizations as the Celiac Disease Foundation and the Gluten Intolerance Group.

With one strong voice, our diversified group sounded the alarm and spread the word about the importance of regulatory standards for gluten-free labeling.

Just as we were arriving at our first meetings, Andrea's phone rang. It was the assistant to Mike Taylor, the deputy commissioner for foods at the FDA, asking whether Deputy Commissioner Taylor could address our group at the cake party that evening. The gluten-free gods were smiling on us.

That evening, Deputy Commissioner Taylor told the crowd: "We will get it done!"

It was two more years before the rule was released in August 2013. But I can't help thinking we still might be waiting for a gluten-free standard for food products if we hadn't built a giant cake and marched to Capitol Hill.

If you ever consider bringing attention to a cause and think it can't be done, bake a cake, bake lots of layers, take a bite, and reflect on how one little band of people on a single mission took on the US government to make life better for millions.

Raising Your GF IQ:
Food-Labeling Regulations

Should I worry when a gluten-free product label says "processed in a factory that also processes wheat products"?

If it also says "gluten-free" on the label, you don't need to worry. Otherwise, you need to have more information before you can make a decision. Manufacturers put a disclaimer on their products for a variety of reasons. Some don't want the liability if someone who is seriously gluten-free becomes ill. Then again, some manufacturers have a policy that requires them to add this disclaimer when, in fact, there is almost no wheat in the plant and it's only used in a section at the opposite end of the facility from where the gluten-free products are made. That tends to minimize the concerns, but you could not know this information without calling the company.

What if one company makes chicken broth, for instance, and makes the "gluten-free" claim, and another makes chicken broth, makes the claim, and adds the warning?

They are both considered gluten-free. If the product label also says "gluten-free" that means it meets the gluten-free standard of less than 20 ppm.

What about the USDA? Does it have any gluten-free regulations?

The USDA regulates meat, poultry, cold cuts, hot dogs, and some egg products, and does not have separate guidelines for wheat, rye, and barley. Most companies voluntarily declare wheat if it is contained in the product. And many are calling out "gluten-free" if their products contain no gluten. The USDA has indicated it will work with the FDA to have consistent labeling on the products it regulates. Meanwhile, if a USDA product label states that it is gluten-free, that does not necessarily mean it contains less than 20 ppm of gluten. Although USDA products that are labeled "gluten-free" are usually safe, the manufacturer is not required to comply with the FDA labeling rule.

Picking Safe Foods

When the FDA regulation came out, someone said to me, "Now I'll know what I can and can't have."

I wish it was that black and white. Yes, we have a great deal more information to help us select safe foods. But gluten-free labeling is voluntary. Some manufacturers who once made the claim may decide not to make it any longer. Others might not say "gluten-free" on their products although the items look safe and probably contain no gluten. It's the manufacturer's choice.

Your best bet is to select products from dedicated gluten-free companies that have a long history with gluten-free consumers. Many have a system in place to vet each supplier and test each batch of product before it is released, or to test frequently.

You should also select products from companies that have third-party certification. These programs establish a protocol with manufacturers before they can be certified and require follow-up testing.

Of course, you can always rely on the naturally gluten-free foods, too—meats, vegetables, dairy, fish, fruits, legumes.

Go with the Pros: Dedicated Companies

"I think the main point that differentiates dedicated gluten-free manufacturers from other companies that make gluten-full and gluten-free products is that the focus for dedicated brands is always about the gluten-free consumer. To these dedicated brands, gluten-free is never an afterthought. It is all we do—it is all we think about. Along with that customer focus is the trust that consumers have in dedicated brands to provide safe products. Without ever reading the label or making sure you picked up the right version, they know, for instance, if it says Glutino or Udi's, it will always be gluten-free."

—LAURA KUYKENDALL,
DIRECTOR OF MARKETING, GLUTINO

Gluten-free Food Pyramid

Imagine the companies that provide our food as a pyramid with tiers indicating the best choices for a person who is seriously gluten-free, safe choices for those who are avoiding gluten by choice, and the areas in between. Unlike the old food pyramid from the USDA, the top tiers of this pyramid are where the safest, risk-free foods reside and the largest areas are the danger zones

Companies at the Top (Dedicated Gluten-free Companies)

Examples: Dr. Schär, Ener-G Foods, Enjoy Life Foods, Glutino, Kinnikinnick, Pamela's Products, Udi's

- Have a long history of making products for people who are seriously gluten-free
- State "gluten-free" on the package
- Manufacture only gluten-free foods
- Likely process products in facilities that do not contain wheat
- Vet their suppliers to prevent cross-contamination issues
- Perform random testing on their products or test every batch before it is released to consumers
- Might also have their products reviewed by an outside gluten-free certification program and carry that symbol on their packaging
- This tier includes naturally gluten-free foods, such as fruits, vegetables, most meats, poultry, fish, and dairy that are nearly always safe, whether they are labeled "gluten-free" or not.

Companies in the Second Tier
(Those with a Strong Commitment to Gluten-free Consumers)

Examples: King Arthur, Betty Crocker, General Mills, Pillsbury

- Mainstream companies that note "gluten-free" on some of their products and therefore meet the FDA standard of less than 20 ppm

- May or may not also use one of the certification programs
- May process in dedicated gluten-free facilities and note it on the label
- Probably have a gluten-free list on their website so you know they've made a commitment to gluten-free consumers
- Perform batch or random testing on products before they go into distribution. Their stake in making this commitment is huge and they know it.

Companies in the Third Tier

Examples: Companies that do not make the gluten-free claim, but product labels don't reveal any obvious gluten-containing ingredients. The labeling might say "no gluten ingredients" but the products do not say "gluten-free."

- The company's level of commitment to gluten-free consumers is not clear. Although the products look like they contain no gluten, these companies have chosen not to include "gluten-free" on their labels, so they are not required to comply with the FDA labeling regulation.
- All manufacturers need to follow FDA Good Manufacturing Practices and thoroughly clean down equipment before manufacturing each product. This might be enough to control cross-contamination.
- Then again, it depends on the product, other products made in the facility, and the company's internal policies about allergen claims.
- Before you eat anything from the gray zone, you might need to call the company's customer service number to get a clearer understanding of their manufacturing process and commitment to gluten-free consumers.
- That's why this is the gray zone.

Companies in the Wide Band of Black at the Bottom

No need to go here. This is the danger zone.

- Products in this band might be labeled "contains wheat," or "may contain traces of wheat." The ingredient label might list one of the other gluten-containing ingredients you need to avoid, such as malt, barley, brewer's yeast, or rye.

How to Use This Pyramid

These lists aren't exhaustive; you'll have to put on your detective hat. Rely primarily on products made by companies that manufacture only gluten-free foods and foods that are naturally gluten-free and by companies that call out "gluten-free" on the product label. Once you've done your research and know which companies you can trust, put those in the top two tiers of your pyramid. If you venture into the gray zone, do so infrequently. Call the manufacturer if you have questions about any product. And stay out of the black zone!

Gluten-free Food Pyramid

People with celiac disease, DH, or gluten sensitivity will want to avoid the Black Zone and eat carefully in the Gray Zone.
Gluten Avoiders can enjoy foods in the 1st, 2nd, and 3rd tiers, but should stay out of the Black Zone.

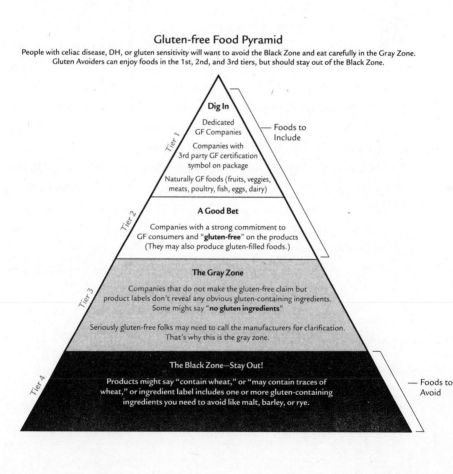

Dig In
Dedicated GF Companies
Companies with 3rd party GF certification symbol on package
Naturally GF foods (fruits, veggies, meats, poultry, fish, eggs, dairy)

Tier 1 — Foods to Include

A Good Bet
Companies with a strong commitment to GF consumers and "**gluten-free**" on the products (They may also produce gluten-filled foods.)

Tier 2

The Gray Zone
Companies that do not make the gluten-free claim but product labels don't reveal any obvious gluten-containing ingredients. Some might say "**no gluten ingredients**"
Seriously gluten-free folks may need to call the manufacturers for clarification. That's why this is the gray zone.

Tier 3

The Black Zone—Stay Out!
Products might say "contain wheat," or "may contain traces of wheat," or ingredient label includes one or more gluten-containing ingredients you need to avoid like malt, barley, or rye.

Tier 4 — Foods to Avoid

Lingering Doubts

The FDA rule may not clear up every question you have about products. Here are some areas where confusion may still lurk.

- The FDA will not be able to monitor every company all the time and most likely will only pursue complaints, which means people have to eat a product to know whether it makes them sick.
- The gluten-free labeling rule is voluntary. A company does not need to use it even if the product contains no gluten and would test well below the 20 ppm threshold. The manufacturers of some products you've been using might not be willing to claim that their products are gluten-free.
- Even if a company chooses to label some of its products, that doesn't mean every product from the company is gluten-free.
- If a product does not contain wheat but is not listed as safe for a gluten-free diet, the company is under no obligation to tell you. It's pretty much up to you.

Shopping Basics

Ever heard the term *shopping the outside aisles*? That's us. The gluten-free shoppers. Stick to foods on the outside aisles of the grocery store, where the basic unprocessed foods reside—fruits, vegetables, meats, and dairy. Nearly all are fresh and they are also naturally gluten-free. They also happen to be healthier.

What's left? The inside aisles, the majority of the store, are filled with processed foods and many contain gluten. That's where you'll also find gluten-free packaged foods—breads, rolls, crackers, cereal, pizza, pasta, and desserts. This is where good label reading is important (see pages 117–118). Thanks to FALCPA and the FDA gluten-free food labeling rule, label reading is easier than it's ever been. But you're not off the hook. You'll need to read labels as you shop. So don't forget your reading glasses.

According to the Bureau of Labor Statistics American Time Use Survey, the average person spends less than forty-five minutes per day shopping for goods and services. But those of us on a gluten-free diet need to allow a little extra time to read labels carefully, especially when we first embark on this diet. (Some people say they spend two hours grocery shopping when they start out.) You'll quickly get the hang of this. Bring along a cup of coffee and download a product app to fortify you (see gluten-free apps, page 311).

The good news is that most of your grocery needs can be met in one visit to the supermarket. You can buy dinner, breakfast, and lunch items and stock up on gluten-free foods at the same time.

Be a Savvy Shopper

Traditionally, stores displayed all their gluten-free products in an 8- or 12-foot section, usually set up in an area labeled "Natural Foods," and devoted a section in the freezer case to gluten-free foods.

Over the past few years, sales of gluten-free foods have grown so much that there are too many products to squeeze into one section of the store. Besides, with roughly one in five Americans selecting gluten-free items, grocers see the monetary benefit of adding more shelf space.

In place of a gluten-free section, gluten-free items are being integrated into the product categories all over the store. Gluten-free mixes are with regular baking mixes, crackers are with gluten-filled crackers. You get the picture. It makes good business sense to get the gluten-free consumer to shop all the aisles. To help them identify the gluten-free items, little gluten-free tags often hang below the appropriate products on the shelves. But it still can be overwhelming. Here are some tips on being a savvy shopper:

- Find out your store's philosophy. Are products integrated throughout the store or does it devote a single area to gluten-free products?
- If the products are integrated into the appropriate sections, does the store keep a list of gluten-free items to help you shop? Suggest this if it doesn't have a list.
- If the products are segregated into one spot, is the section labeled? Ask a customer service person to direct you.

- A channel marker is the ticket that slides into the front edge of the shelf where a product lives. It includes the price, bar code for the item, and the name of the product. Below or attached to this ticket should be another tag that calls out "gluten-free."
- Keep in mind that you are in the hands of the stock person who set up the shelves and the buyer who orders the items and that not everyone shares your understanding of the gluten-free category.
- Integrated products are not always marked correctly.
- Things move. The product and its tags should reside in an assigned space. But one product sells out and, before the reorder arrives, a stock person or customer moves the next door neighbor into that space. It happens all the time. And this product might not be gluten-free even if the tag on the shelf says "gluten-free." Look at the channel marker and make sure the product on the shelf matches the item on the ticket.
- Products look similar. If a company makes a gluten-free and a gluten-filled line of products, it may use the same design for both, varying colors slightly and adding a gluten-free banner to one set of packaging. Now that many products sit side by side, it's easy to grab the wrong one. And some may be labeled "wheat-free" but are not gluten-free.
- Double-check labels. Ingredients change. Companies may change the gluten-free status of the product, too. Read each product before you purchase it to make sure it is, indeed, gluten-free.

Saving Money—Shop the Sales

Who doesn't like a bargain, especially when it comes to gluten-free food? Here are ways to get the most bang for your buck:

- When an item goes on sale or you have a couple of coupons, grab extras and store them in the freezer.
- If a favorite food company offers free shipping (online) or discounts, that's the time to load up and freeze extras.
- Buying in bulk can save money, too, as long as you have space to store it.

For more on saving money see page 287.

If you are new to the GFD, you might feel as if you are saying good-bye to great breads, pizza, doughnuts, and the like. Not so. Today, you'll find great gluten-free counterparts for just about everything you've given up. Browse the middle aisles of the supermarket and you'll discover cereals, pasta, cookies, crackers, and more. In the freezer section, you'll see an assortment of cakes, cookies, muffins, and bread. Yes, and even the bread is pretty decent.

Gut Reaction: The Big Chew—A History of Bread

The first time I was diagnosed with celiac disease as a young child, I ate a lot of bananas—fried, mashed with dates, wrapped in Canadian bacon and broiled. Indeed, it was a strange but fascinating menu. I ate broiled steak, cottage cheese, and all the butter I wanted. But there was no bread.

The word *gluten* was never mentioned. But, for more than three years, no starches or sugar came across my plate. Gradually potatoes, corn, rice, and wheat reappeared. About that time I was pronounced "cured."

Fast-forward to when I was twenty-two and traveling in Europe. I fell in love with brioche, Brötchen, and croissant. Dipping hard rolls in café au lait, slathering sweet butter and homemade jam on rich brioche, this was yummyness to the third power.

Back in the USA, I signed on with two roommates in a walkup on Beacon Hill in Boston. Every Friday, one of them baked whole wheat bread. Walking across the Boston Common with a damp chill at my back, I couldn't wait to reach our apartment, where I was greeted by a burst of steam from the oven and the aroma of freshly baked bread. We cut the bread thickly and draped one side with butter and fresh honey. I ate with a gluten frenzy, as if this might be my last slice of bread. Little did I know.

In 1976, I was rediagnosed. These two memories of bread lingered in my culinary DNA, but it would be years until I found a gluten-free

▶

bread that approximated the chew and taste of the real stuff that filled my days in Europe and on Beacon Hill.

Until then, the big chew was gone. I was facing a gluten unload.

The gluten-free breads in 1976 were filled with methylcellulose; they looked like bread and held their shape. But biting into a slice was like chewing on a Styrofoam cup. No amount of toasting or jam or honey could mask that unmistakable texture. My gut told me I would never eat bread again. But one day in the early eighties, I discovered a European company that was importing a gluten-free bread mix into the United States. It rose like a real bread. It filled the kitchen with a tantalizing aroma and domed like a genuine loaf. I was giddy with excitement. Bread was back—well, almost.

I lopped off a hunk from one end. Slathered it in butter and honey. The texture wasn't quite like Beacon Hill whole wheat bread, but after nearly a decade without, it was pretty decent. How had this company been able to ditch the Styrofoam texture? What was its secret?

Among the ingredients listed on the sterile-looking box, was something called xanthan gum. Along with its cousin guar gum, these would become a critical element in putting the chew back in gluten-free baking, adding back some of the elasticity that is synonymous with gluten. Manufacturers had been using it for years in everything from ice cream to chewing gum, and now these gums were available in consumer-size packages for gluten-free bakers who were discovering that a pinch lends structure to dough, allows the yeast to rise, and produces nearly normal loaves.

It took manufacturers (most of which did not have to eat gluten-free) years to figure out the nuances of baking with gums. If a little was good, a lot was better. The early breads had jaw-breaking chewiness. A person could maw on a single bite for hours. Fortified with memories of real breads and a package of xanthan gum, I became an expert on gluten-free bread. I began Gluten-free Pantry in 1993, offering the best gluten-free bread possible. For many years my Favorite Sandwich Bread was the top-selling bread among gluten-free people. Favorite Sandwich Bread raised the bar—up over the rim of the pan and into a beautifully domed loaf.

▼

Today, with the huge growth in gluten-free products and desire to capture a share of that market, manufacturers are hard at work to build a better bread. Several years ago, Udi's raised the bar a little higher, blanketing the country with its breads, rolls, and bagels. Then Glutino added another light-textured prepared bread. Rudi's, Nature's Path, Canyon Bake House, Dr. Schär, and Kinnikinnick soon joined the bread lines with competing products. And artisan bakers added freshly baked choices and more whole grains.

As the bread wars heat up, it's good news for consumers who reap the benefits of manufacturer endeavors. We all win and the prize is a slice of the big chew.

Separating the Wheat from the Chaff: Communion Wafers

The wildest misconception I've heard is people who tell me, "The Communion wafer has been blessed by Jesus. It can't make me sick."

—ANNE ROLAND LEE, EdD, RD, LD, DIRECTOR OF
NUTRITIONAL SERVICES FOR DR. SCHÄR USA AND A
REGISTERED DIETITIAN WHO WORKS WITH CELIAC DISEASE PATIENTS

The Communion Conundrum

With all due respect, there are some things that heart and head cannot control. Regular Communion wafers contain wheat and will still give a celiac or gluten-sensitive person tummy trouble. In addition, if ingested every week, this can surely wreak havoc on the gut and your antibodies.

For parishioners who participate in religions where Holy Communion is part of the regular church service, the host and wine are links to spiritual fulfillment and a gluten conundrum. Until recently, the Catholic

Church required Communion wafers be made with wheat in order to be consecrated. But recently the Vatican deemed that "low-gluten wafers may be used at Mass in the United States with appropriate permission."

Benedictine Sisters of Perpetual Adoration stepped in and now make Vatican-approved low-gluten Communion wafers, using some wheat starch but registering less than 20 ppm of gluten. They are not harmful to most celiac and gluten-sensitive people but fulfill the requirements of the Church. Purchase these through the Benedictine Sisters of Perpetual Adoration, 1-800-223-2772 or e-mail altarbreads@benedictinesisters.org.

Gluten-free Communion Wafers

For denominations that allow a gluten-free alternative, Ener-G Foods offers Communion wafers that contain no wheat. Although they are not consecrated, these gluten-free hosts are approved by the Evangelical Lutheran Church in America, the Episcopal Church, and the United Methodist Church. Go to ener-g.com.

People who are gluten-free by choice and participate in regular Communion at a Catholic church may want to purchase low-gluten wafers, depending on how strictly they are following a GFD.

Children and Cross-Contamination

First Communion is a special time for a child and his or her family. But it becomes challenging when the child about to make First Communion is also a child who cannot have gluten. Today the availability of low-gluten Communion wafers makes it easier. But the issue of cross-contamination is still a concern. Talk with the priest who will be leading the Mass that day and devise a way to set your child's wafer apart. Using a separate plate marked with the child's name works well. In addition, ask the priest to let your child go first so the chalice of wine is not cross-contaminated from others who have eaten the regular Host.

Adults and older children will want to apply these tips to avoid cross-contamination when they take Communion, too.

You Don't Have to Be
Jewish to Enjoy Passover

For several weeks prior to Passover, stores begin stocking kosher for Passover pastries, noodles, mixes, and rice- or oat-based matzo. This is the start of a shopping frenzy for gluten-free people who stockpile treats as if they are preparing for their own Exodus. And here's why. Foods for Passover cannot contain any wheat, barley, rye, or spelt. The exception is matzo and matzo meal, the unleavened form of wheat, which are used in some Passover products. Those will say "contains wheat" on the label. But most Passover foods are safe. These products must be produced in facilities that are free from any wheat contamination in accordance with kosher for Passover standards. Rather than cleaning the plant to rid it of every crumb of *chametz* (the forbidden grains) in accordance with stringent Passover dietary laws, companies often keep separate facilities just to make Passover foods. In fact, the Passover products have become so popular with gluten-free folks that several manufacturers now produce their Passover line year-round. Tip: Look for products labeled "non-*gebrockts*." That lets you know they contain no matzo.

All Things Deli

No matter how you slice it, anyone who follows a gluten-free diet, whether it's for medical reasons or a lifestyle choice, will want to read this section before his or her next trip to the deli counter. Here's some basic deli-intelligence.

You've probably noticed that many brands of deli meat now make the gluten-free claim. That's great news, but truthfully, I wonder how many were always safe and only took notice about the time the gluten-free frenzy caught hold. Such companies as Boar's Head and Dietz and Watson paved the way by responding to the celiac community's inquiries several years ago. And today, it seems as if new brands touting "gluten-free" on their labels appear every time I visit the deli counter.

Only a couple of areas bear warning. Most hams, for instance, are gluten-free, although the glaze on some whole ham products can contain wheat.

And you'll want to watch out for highly processed deli meats, such as pressed loaves, where scraps of meat and by-products are "welded" into shape by using binders and broths. Turkey roll, meat loaf, liverwurst, and pepper loaf fall into this category. (Speaking of processed meats, sausages and hot dogs are iffy, too, as some use fillers and flavorings, such as bread crumbs, soy sauce, and liquid smoke.) And occasionally roast beef can be injected with flavorings that contain gluten. The folks at the deli counters can show you the ingredient list for each product. Read that list before purchasing or stick with products that are labeled "gluten-free."

And while meats and poultry do not fall under the gluten-free food labeling rule, the companies making the gluten-free claim on their deli meats are major corporations and not likely to do so unless they already meet the FDA standard.

Not every product from every company is gluten-free, however; again, double-check before purchasing. Usually the gluten-free items will be listed on the company websites, too. (See Resources, page 313, for a list of gluten-free deli brands.)

Deli Counter Concerns: Shared Equipment

I don't think cold cuts, as a rule, should be a major concern for people who cannot have gluten. But what about shared equipment? Some stores have a dedicated slicer for all gluten-free deli meats. I love that. Conversely, some folks are afraid to order deli in a place that does not have a dedicated slicer. I am not sure that degree of worry is necessary. To begin with, very few deli products contain gluten. But ask the person serving you to change his or her gloves and discard the first slice in your order, just for peace of mind.

One source does worry me and it's not the actual slicer. Some delis prepare sandwiches at the same counter where they slice all the cold cuts and that spells cross-contamination, big time. Watch what's going on and determine for yourself whether sandwiches are made in the same area where the meats are sliced. If they are on top of one another, find another place to purchase cold cuts. Or purchase prepackaged cold cuts. Many brands make the "gluten-free" claim on the package. And, of course, if your deli counter offers gluten-free sandwiches, be sure they are made in a clean area, using clean utensils.

Raising Your GF IQ: Maybe It's GF—but Do You Really Want to Eat That Stuff?

Is pink slime safe for a gluten-free diet?

Unfortunately, pink slime, also known as finely textured ground beef, is gluten-free. Pink slime is ammonium hydroxide–treated beef (well, actually beef parts that I will not detail here). Often listed as "finely textured ground beef," this is responsible for giving ground beef that lovely red color that makes it look forever fresh.

But tree bark, slugs, and snakes are gluten-free, too. Who wants to eat them?

Let's you and me have a private little talk between these pages. You are now being mindful of what you eat gluten-wise. Don't you think you might want to be more mindful of the rest of your diet, too? Some things just should not be and this is one of them.

What is meat glue and is it gluten-free?

Here's another one. Some call it meat glue; officially, it is known as transglutaminase (eTG), and it's another food additive. Like ammonium hydroxide, it's unlikely to be found on product labels. Meat glue is used to bind pieces of meat and fish and keeps liquids from separating in such things as yogurt and ice cream.

In the book *Celiac Disease: A Hidden Epidemic*, by Peter H. R. Green, MD, and Rory Jones, transglutaminase (eTG) is described as "part of an arsenal of additives that enable food manufacturers to increase the texture, shelf life and appearance of their products. While it is unknown how widely this enzyme is used, a recent study done in the Netherlands showed that eating food treated with eTG can enhance the immune response of people with celiac disease."[2]

Let's be honest: this topic scares me. There is no way to know when a food contains transglutaminase. Use of this and other additives makes me want to retreat (no, run) to the outside aisles of the supermarket, where I can shop for fresh, unprocessed food.

And making great meals by incorporating safe commercial gluten-free products, healthy fruits, vegetables, meats, and dairy and a little culinary ingenuity is not as difficult as you'd think. That's coming next.

9

Your GF-Friendly Kitchen

Whether you are setting up a dedicated gluten-free kitchen or sharing it with gluten-eaters, this section will help you get started, know the pitfalls (where gluten can hide) and the ways to please gluten eaters and gluten-free folks without feeling like you've become a short order cook. If you have celiac disease or gluten sensitivity, please read every crumb of this section. If you are gluten-free by choice, the choice is yours. Only you know the degree of vigilance you bring to this diet. But do me a favor and at least skim this chapter. Even if you don't need this level of gluten awareness, you probably have friends who do and will eat in your home one day.

Surprising Places Where Gluten Lurks: Kitchen Cross-Contamination

When gluten mingles with gluten-free food, there's a real chance that a gluten-free person can have a reaction that's not unlike eating wheat, itself. Common sources of contamination include eating and cooking utensils, cups, dishware, hands, aprons, Teflon-coated pans, colanders, countertops, and cooling racks. But here are some others that might surprise you.

Bread Machine

As its name implies, the bread machine makes bread. Lots of potential gluten here. If you share the machine, clean the paddles, and the neck where they attach, very carefully—gluteny dough can get caught in these small crevices.

Remedy: Buy a second bread pan and paddles. The machine itself never touches the dough. Label one "GF" and put a skull and crossbones on the other.

Charcoal Briquettes and Wheat

Believe it or not, charcoal briquettes can contain wheat. Many are made of a composite of materials, including wheat starch. The jury is out on whether the wheat can actually get into your food. The coals should be white when the grill is ready. Some think the wheat has burned off. Others worry about the ash flying into their food.

Remedy: To be on the safe side, grill with hardwood charcoal, or better yet, use a gas grill.

Can Opener

Gone are the days when every can lid had to be cranked open. But still a good portion of our canned foods require a can opener to get at the contents. I would give the lecture about not using so many canned products but, hey, I get that you have a busy household.

I also get that you have a teenager whose after-school snack every day is canned ravioli in a thick tomato sauce. And the next kid in line, the middle school child, has celiac disease and likes canned gluten-free chicken and rice soup with gluten-free crackers for his snack.

So number one kid opens the ravioli and hands the can opener to number two child, who then opens his can of soup and smears a thick streak of gluteny tomato sauce over the rim of the can. Cross-contamination? You betcha.

Remedy: Buy an extra can opener and label it with a big "GF."

Cast-Iron Skillets

Cast iron is not as much of a problem as Teflon, which can develop deep scratches where gluten can linger (see "Teflon-Coated Cookware," page 147), but the material is porous and can retain gluten if not carefully cleaned.

Remedy: Run cast-iron skillets and griddles through the dishwasher and then season them again. Keep these for gluten-free cooking only. It's a bother to clean them properly every time someone wants regular pancakes.

Condiments: Butter, Jelly, Peanut Butter

These are three musketeers of mischief. They are close friends with bread, toast, rolls, biscuits, and scones, and someone is going to get into trouble if they are shared. One member of the family, a gluten-full person, comes along and dips a knife into the grape jelly, then smears it on a piece of toast, then goes back for more using the same knife or scrapes the leftover jelly back into the jar. The gluten-free person comes along next and decides he wants grape jelly on his gluten-free toast. He dips his knife in the same jar and gets more than just grape jelly. He gets gluten crumbs, too. A small amount might not cause a detectable reaction, but day after day, this practice can cause the gluten-free person to get pretty sick.

Ditto for butter and peanut butter containers. This trio of condiments are harbingers of bad news.

Remedy: Don't let these musketeers duke it out. If this is a blended household, keep separate jars of peanut butter, jelly, and sticks of butter and label them so there is no concern about cross-contamination. Here's where stickers work well.

Convection Oven

A convection oven circulates the air evenly throughout the oven by means of a system of powerful fans. These are terrific for baking, but no friend to the gluten-free baker. For one thing, the blowing air pushes gluten-free doughs into all sorts of weird shapes: pointy, droopy hats on muffins and cupcakes, and cookies with rippled molten lava–looking tops. For another, if you bake gluten and gluten-free in the same oven, some of the flour particles are guaranteed to comingle as they blow around. This is a breeding ground for disaster.

Remedy: Avoid using the convection setting on your oven except to cook nonpastry items and *never* bake gluten and gluten-free stuff on the convection setting at the same time. If you do a lot of gluten-filled baking, wipe down the oven carefully (even use the "clean" cycle) before you bake gluten-free foods. Ideally, invest in a separate portable oven if you do a lot of both kinds of baking.

Cutlery Drawer

This drawer gets more use than a roll of toilet paper. If you don't believe me, just count the number of times you open that drawer for a spoon, a fork, or a knife. And there's your teenage son with a piece of toast in one hand and the other rummaging for a knife, while your toddler drools animal cracker juice into the drawer as she rests her chin on the edge so she can peer in and find a sippy straw.

Remedy: Clean the drawer often and keep munchers and munchkins away from this territory.

Cutting Board

The cutting board, too, sees a lot of action—breads, sandwiches, English muffins, pizza are all cut and sliced here. If the gluten-free varieties are also prepared on this surface, you're certain to add a few crumbs of gluten to your food.

Remedy: Designate separate cutting boards for gluten and gluten-free, particularly if the board is wooden, as it may be difficult to clean the surface thoroughly. If the board is plastic, wash it carefully before preparing gluten-free items.

Flour Sifter

If you used this prediagnosis, throw it away. It is difficult to clean out all the residual flour.

Remedy: Buy two separate sifters and label for future use.

Food Processors

Dough creeps into the shaft of the blades and it hardens. Then it cracks and flakes into your gluten-free mixture. *Ewww.* Although this machine has fewer places for gluten to hide than does the mixer or bread machine, it's challenging to scrub every nook and cranny to a pristine cleanliness.

Remedy: Keep a second set of blades or a separate processor for gluten-free preparations.

Grill

Bread crumbs from toasting hamburger rolls, residual barbecue sauce that contains wheat, grilled pizza . . . all of these can leave a trail of gluten. And you know what happens next: that gluten's transferred to the next item and that could be yours.

Remedy: Preheat the grill so that any residual food burns off. Then brush the grids carefully before grilling your food. To be extra safe, grill on a sheet of aluminum foil spread over the heated grids. Go first before anyone has had a chance to contaminate the grill.

Im-Pasta-Bility

Pasta leaches gluten into the water as it cooks and onto the colander when it is drained.

Remedy: Use a separate pot and colander when preparing gluten-free and gluten-filled pasta. Be careful not to use the same spoons to mix sauces into gluten-containing pasta and then into gluten-free pasta. This, too, can be a source of cross-contamination.

Additional tips: Gluten is removed from most pots and colander when they are washed in the dishwasher. But who has time to wash a colander while making dinner? If you drain and remove the gluten-free pasta first, you need only one. If you don't have a dishwasher, you'll need to be more mindful when cleaning gluteny contents from a colander or strainer, and slotted spoons and spatulas, too, for that matter. Consider keeping two sets of these and label one so it never touches gluten.

Gluten-free pasta has become so tasty and affordable that you might not need two kinds any more. Most people can't tell the difference, especially in lasagna recipes (see page 185 for a GF recipe).

Mixer

Dough creeps into the crevices where the beaters lock into the mixer head. No matter how hard you try, it's difficult to scrub everything to a pristine cleanliness. But making matters worse, when the dough hardens, it cracks and the vibration from the motor causes it to flake off into your gluten-free dough. Gross, huh?

Remedy: Keep a second mixer or use yours only for gluten-free baking.

Pet Food

Kids like to share, whether it's the dog's treats, the kibble, or the fish food. Unless your pet is on a gluten-free diet, too, most of the pet food you bring home probably contains wheat. And when you feed the animals, the fallout—on the counter, food particles flying onto a sandwich—can be downright contaminating to an unsuspecting gluten-free person.

Don't be tempted by chic new grain-free and gluten-free dog foods that might not be either. Even if the ingredients sound safe, who knows how they've been manufactured.

Remedy: Put Fido and his food in the doghouse. Pick one safe area to feed pets where toddlers are not playing and away from the kitchen, where gluten can land on food and counters. Watch out for fish food, too. Those little wafers can hold a day's worth of misery.

Sponges

Sponges are a breeding ground for bacteria. You wipe a surface with a wet sponge and it picks up little crumbs of food that stick to the sponge and breed like cells in a petri dish. If you wipe a flour-coated surface with a sponge, you are breeding more than bugs. You are moving the flour to places where the gluten-free person's food is prepared. If you wash a bowl that's coated with leftover oatmeal or bread dough, that's going to cling, too.

Remedy: Designate one color sponge (dish and counter) for gluten and one for gluten-free. Use paper towels to wipe up gluteny messes or wipe out gluten-filled dishes. (This goes for dishrags, pot-scrubber pads, and scrub brushes, too.)

Teflon-Coated Cookware

Teflon pans can get deep scratches that reduce the nonstick capabilities and provide a place where gluten can hang around for a long time.

Remedy: Either separate out your pots and pans or use stainless-steel (or cast-iron) cookware, which is easy to wash. If your cookware has rivets on the inside surface to hold the handle in place, make sure to clean those surfaces carefully as particles of gluten can get trapped there, too.

Toaster

What is a toaster's primary function? That's right. It's to toast bread. Could there be a greater ticking time bomb in the house? Between residual wheat that attaches to the grids and wheat crumbs sprinkling into the bottom of the toaster, this little appliance has the potential to be one of the biggest sources of cross-contamination.

Remedy: Many people keep a separate toaster to use for their gluten-free bread. Others clean carefully after a family member has toasted *real* bread. A toaster oven presents a little less risk, as the grid is horizontal and easy to access and clean. The crumbs fall into a tray that can be removed and cleaned. And the tray is nicely tucked away so it never comes into contact with your gluten-free toast. Or use a toaster bag to toast gluten-free bread and protect your toast from gluten crumbs (see page 222).

Raising Your GF IQ: Myths About Kitchen Cross-Contamination

Gluten cannot be washed off pots and pans.

Most smooth surfaces can be safely cleaned with soap and water. The exceptions are porous materials, such as cast iron and Teflon (see pages 143 and 147). And don't share wooden cutting boards, either.

It's okay to store gluten-free and gluten-filled foods in the same cabinets and drawers.

Yes and no. If these are in separate, sealed packages or resealable plastic bags and marked to indicate which ones are gluten-free, you should be fine. But no comingling, please. Storing an open box of gluten-free crackers in the same plastic bag with gluten-filled crackers is dangerous. As if cross-contamination wasn't enough of a concern, the original packaging can become separated from the food and you'll never know for certain which are the safe crackers and which ones will send you to the bathroom. For best protection, designate shelves gluteny and gluten-free.

Paper towels contain gluten.

Paper towels are a friend to people on a GFD. They are great for reheating food, keeping a layer of protection between your food and the microwave if it's shared, and a safe way to wipe out dishes and utensils if the sponge might be contaminated. The sheets of paper are perfectly safe. There are some reports that a layer of glue used to hold the last sheet on the roll may contain gluten. I always discard that sheet just to be safe. Besides it's gunked up with glue and kind of disgusting.

Paper plates and plastic utensils are not safe.

There's no truth to the rumor that these contain gluten. After much research, I could not find a single one that is gluten-based.

Toasters are okay. The gluten burns off.

Toasters are not okay for several reasons (see "Toaster," page 147) But what about the issue about gluten's being burned off? It's a nice thought, but not likely. The surface needs to be washed to remove gluten.

Flour in the air won't hurt.

Technically that's true, unless you have a wheat allergy. But if I am in a bakery for too long, my mouth starts to feel funny. Maybe I mouth breath too much, but it seems to me that airborne flour can find its way to the mouth. Don't take a chance. Besides, what are you doing in a bakery, anyway? There's nothing safe to eat here. And if a bakery offers one or two gluten-free items, those aren't likely to be safe either (again, think about all that gluten flying around . . .).

It's okay to bake a regular pizza and gluten-free pizza together.

I don't recommend it, but if you do this, make sure the gluten-free pizza is on a rack above the gluten-filled pizza so anything that shakes off either pan floats to the bottom of the oven. Truthfully, you might want to consider baking these separately, baking the gluten-free pizza first and never baking gluten and gluten-free in a convection oven.

Dishwashing detergent contains gluten.

No, these do not contain gluten.

Household cleaners contain gluten, so they should be avoided.

I wish that was true. I could excuse myself from a lot of household chores. But most do not contain gluten, and even if they did, I doubt you would be ingesting any of these products, right?! If you worry about using a product on the kitchen counters where you handle food, wipe the area with a damp paper towel after you clean. The same with pots and pans and silverware. Who wants cleaning chemicals touching food, anyway? And you can always rely on white vinegar and baking soda as your primary cleaning materials and keep the chemicals out entirely.

Bleach and disinfectant are the only way to get rid of gluten.
Gluten is a protein, not a bacteria. No need to dig out the antibacterial cleansers. But you will need to scrub surfaces with soap and water. So put the Lysol away and get out the elbow grease.

A Blended (Diet) Family

So, the doctor put your son on a gluten-free diet. Do you need to make everyone in the family go gluten-free? Or is it okay to make separate meals? Does the risk of cross-contamination outweigh trying to keep gluten in the house?

Most of us live in blended-diet families. One or two eat gluten-free; the others eat everything or are just plain picky. You didn't sign on to be a short-order cook and you don't need to be one now.

Making sure food is safe for the person who needs a gluten-free diet is priority number one. But consider this. Most of the basics in meal preparation—meat, fish, vegetables, fruit, and dairy—is already gluten-free. Make these the foundation for your meal planning.

If you serve bread, this is where you can add gluten-free and gluten-filled options. And make sure they are cut with separate knives on separate cutting boards and served on separate plates. The same is true for desserts. Ice cream and fruit are great communal options. (Some ice cream contains pretzels, cookie dough, or brownie crumbs. Read the labels before serving.)

On taco night, serve fillings everyone can eat and place flour and corn tortillas in separate baskets. Be careful not to comingle the serving utensils. When the family eats pizza, choose a gluten-free variety for the folks who need it and serve regular pizza for those who don't. Be careful not to share the pizza wheel or knife. And serve gluten-free chicken nuggets (many affordably priced brands are available) and dipping sauce to the whole family.

There's no one-size-fits-all when it comes to folding special diets into family meals but by keeping the basics safe for all and adding gluten-free and gluten-filled choices where appropriate, you can make it easy to keep everyone happy.

I asked others who juggle gluteny and gluten-free diets to weigh in on this subject and the majority said they make one meal for everyone. That's especially true when the primary cook is the person who needs a gluten-free diet or when more than one person needs to eat this way. Or as one friend says, "My wife is gluten-free. That means we are all on the diet. She just substitutes gluten-free ingredients in all the recipes. I get enough gluten when I go out of town."

And many people do everything the same except for substituting gluten-free pasta, hamburger buns, and sometimes taco shells, because the extra cost of gluten-free food is tough on the food budget.

**"I'm Gluten-free and I'm the Cook.
They Eat What I Make and I Make It Gluten-free."**

Whatever way you choose to incorporate gluten-free foods into family meals, know that your style of blending the family might change as you adapt to this dietary regimen, as the children grow and as new products become available.

Setting Up Your Kitchen

The degree to which you need a gluten-free zone in your kitchen depends on how many people are sharing the kitchen, their ages, and the amount of gluten-filled items used on a daily basis.

The risk of cross-contamination is probably highest in a busy household with young children. Place gluten-containing foods up high and out of reach of youngsters who need a gluten-free diet. Designate one low cupboard for gluten-free treats and label it so everyone, including the youngsters, knows this food is safe. Do the same for gluten-containing treats if children are old enough to understand the rules.

Turn separating and labeling foods into a game. Let each child pick stickers that represent a color or an animal that is his or her favorite. When items are unpacked from the grocery store, give each one the products that are appropriate and let them put stickers on the packages and place them in the cupboard that also bears their sticker and name.

This system works well when grandparents and sitters are helping out, too. Even if they don't understand the diet, they understand the stickers.

As kids get older, they can take more responsibility for choosing and labeling products as well as picking safe foods from the kitchen for snacks and meals. They might still like the stickers, however. It becomes a family affair if everyone participates.

In our home, we eat mostly gluten-free food. My husband eats only cereal and bread that are gluten-filled and draws a skull and crossbones on them so I know they are my poison. (We are kids at heart.) When my son was growing up, I always had homemade bread and rolls in the freezer for his lunches. I made a batch of fresh pasta and froze it in portion-size bags for our dinners. But before you hand me the Suzy Homemaker award, remember this was the nineties. Very few commercial gluten-free products were available and most were not very tasty.

Life is much easier when it's adults only. You can work together to set down a few ground rules that make your blended kitchen a safe kitchen. This includes reminding your partner or roommates not to double dip in the mayo and the peanut butter. It might also mean that you eat only gluten-free at home or that you store gluten-filled foods on one side of the kitchen and gluten-free items on the opposite side. The toaster might continue to be an issue. Either buy a separate one or use a toaster oven that can be easily cleaned of gluten residue.

10

Meals, Cooking, and Baking

We prepare nearly 1,100 meals each calendar year (365 x 3). Add the challenge of cooking and baking everything gluten-free and menu planning can be daunting, especially if you are just embarking on this journey.

Relax. Begin with a few safe choices. A meal can be as simple as a bowl of cereal, a sandwich or a plate of chicken nuggets and they come in your size—gluten-free. These days, there are as many gluten-free foods and ideas as opportunities to eat them. You'll quickly branch out, even do some baking and maybe try your hand at from-scratch recipes.

Let's get started. Here are some tips to help you imagine the possibilities.

1. Eat mainly fruits, vegetables, low-fat protein, whole gluten-free grains, legumes, olive oil, and perhaps a little wine. These are healthy and inherently gluten-free.
2. Celebrate equal opportunity holidays and get-togethers. Serve *the same* (gluten-free) stuffing, pies, cakes, pasta, and gravy to everyone.
3. Include both gluten-filled and gluten-free options in a meal *only* when you must (because of cost or big taste difference, as in breads and rolls).

Breakfast

Breakfast foods are abundant. Gluten-free breads, rolls, and bagels are sold by several companies. (You'll find them in the freezer section, along with English muffins, doughnuts, pancakes, and waffles.) Look for hot and cold cereals, from sugary to whole grain, in supermarkets and natural food stores. If gluten-free oats are tolerated, these, too, come in a variety of flakes (thick, steel-cut, and quick) as well as instant choices. Many brands of yogurt are gluten-free. Just watch out for brands with granola or crunchy cereal on top. And eggs are always fine.

Lunch: Bring Your Own

Some people say that lunch is the most challenging meal. Perhaps that's because it's often the make-and-take meal of the day. To play it safe, many folks take their lunch. It may not be sexy to carry a tote bag to work, but it sure beats getting sick or struggling to find a safe eatery near the office every day. And you have lots of options here, too. Going without sandwiches is a thing of the past, thanks to all the wonderful gluten-free rolls, breads, and wraps available. At least a dozen companies distribute frozen, prepared gluten-free breads nationally and several make wraps from corn or gluten-free flours (see the list on page 313).

Pack gluten-free deli meat, a tomato, and condiments and bread or roll and make a sandwich. If you pack the ingredients separately, the bread doesn't get soggy before lunch time.

Refrigeration is nice, but a cold pack and a thermal lunch bag will do the trick if the refrigerator is gross or nonexistent.

Pack a salad in a large container, but don't dress the salad until you are ready to eat

Bring leftovers from last night's dinner and reheat in a microwave, or bring a can of soup (many are labeled "gluten-free"). Pick cans with pop-top lids rather than cans that require a can opener (for convenience and to minimize cross-contamination).

Bring a frozen pizza or single-serve frozen meal (Amy's and Gluten-freeda are good sources) and heat it at your office.

Office Cross-Contamination

This is one place where co-workers comingle and the results can be ugly. As in your own kitchen, workplace condiment jars and appliances can be teaming with gluten. Even sponges and dish towels—icky. Unlike in your own kitchen, you may not be able to control it!

If you leave your stash in the office kitchen, there is no telling what will happen. Be self-sufficient. Bring salad dressing in a personal-size container. Take single-serving packets of condiments. Line the microwave with paper towels before using it. And avoid the communal toaster at all cost.

Packing School Lunches

This requires a sandwich prep-ahead. But consider the elements. Some breads turn crumbly and others turn soggy. Some products hold up well if they are toasted. Experiment. These need to hold up to your standards as well as to your child's scrutiny.

I've had the best luck with rolls, the least success with wraps. Mayonnaise, mustard, tomatoes, or pickles on do-ahead sandwiches can cause the bread to become soggy, but a slice or two of cheese, if tolerated, adds some flavor and moisture without contributing to the sog factor.

Single-serve pretzels, crackers, corn chips, potato chips, or other gluten-free snack foods and gluten-free granola bars make great additions to kid lunches. GoPicnic, a healthy, gluten-free version of Lunchables, makes great lunch options for kids (adults, too). A thermos of warm soup or chili holds up well and kids welcome the treat when the weather turns cool.

Everyone loves a home-baked treat. This effort is not lost on most kids when it comes to lunch-box cuisine. The sight of a homemade brownie or cookie might have all their classmates drooling with envy. (See "School Lunch," page 238, for tips on setting up a lunch plan with school personnel.)

Tip: Let the kids help shop for additions to their school lunches so they have sanctioned the choices and picked the ones that get the highest approval rating with them and their friends. Besides, this way you can help them pick healthy choices, too. And if a classmate has life-threatening food allergies (e.g., peanuts), you can steer your child away from foods containing that allergen.

Dinner

Dinner can be as simple as dressing up plain meats and fish by adding flavorful marinades or sauces (e.g., chimichurri sauce for pork; barbecue sauce for chicken; and roasted Thai chili paste and lime for fish). Or you can make over stews, casseroles, lasagna, and other one-pot meals by simply replacing the gluteny items with gluten-free ingredients.

Sides, too, require just a bit of substitution ingenuity. Use gluten-free pasta in all your favorite pasta dishes. The taste is very good and competitively priced brands are now available (Barilla and Sam Mills are two). Corn pasta (or a blend of corn and rice) is best for dishes that will be reheated and for pasta salads. (Don't dress pasta salads too far ahead of serving or the noodles will begin to break down and become soggy.) Risotto (made with arborio rice) is naturally gluten-free, but be sure the broth is, too. Add mushrooms, sausage, and cheese, if you like.

As the Mediterranean diet suggests, veggies are our friends. Most vegetables are great for roasting. This technique produces intense flavor and makes you look like a gourmet chef. Cut the veggies and toss with olive oil and kosher salt. Spread on a baking sheet and bake at 425°F until veggies are fork tender and the edges are slightly browned. Potatoes and sweet potatoes are great this way, too. Add roasted veggies to salads or pasta salads. Or think: appetizer, and serve roasted asparagus with a mayonnaise–lemon zest dip for nibbles. How great is that? And simple, too.

Managing Meals with Kids: No One Gets Points for Perfection

Let's face it, if it was you or me, we'd make do with whatever was in the fridge. But juggling kids' routines, a special diet or two, and your own agenda requires a bit more planning. Here are some tricks to take some of the heat off your shoulders without putting it back on the rest of the family. Add your own notes in the margins of these pages or add sticky notes as you find more items.

Kids' parties and playdates also require additional planning; you'll find lots of suggestions and coping skills starting on page 231 of the part on lifestyle.

Quick Meals and Snacks Everyone Will Eat

Use the following as the basis for your own creations or let the kids customize concoctions from a selection of gluten-free choices you have on hand. Most important, have fun!

CHICKEN NUGGETS

- Many affordable gluten-free brands are available. Put your creativity to work making the dipping sauces.

CORN TORTILLAS
(NOT JUST FOR TACOS, BUT BE SURE TO PICK
BRANDS YOU KNOW ARE GLUTEN-FREE)

- Quesadilla. Sandwich two tortillas with cheese and meat. Heat in a skillet to make a quick quesadilla.
- Pizza. Top tortillas with pizza sauce and cheese for instant pizza.
- Inside-Out Pizza. Sandwich pizza toppings between two tortillas and heat in a skillet. Slice into wedges. Dip in pizza sauce.
- Roll-ups. Warm wraps briefly until pliable. Smear with hummus or mayonnaise; add gluten-free deli meat and roll; or cover with peanut or almond butter and banana slices.

GO YOGURT

- Yogurt Swirl. Swirl preserves, fruit, or berries into plain yogurt. Top with nuts, or more fresh fruit. Add a little gluten-free cereal or granola for crunch. For a special treat, freeze the mixture for about 30 minutes.
- Chocolate Parfait. Drizzle chocolate sauce into plain or flavored yogurt. Top with mini-marshmallows and chocolate bits.

- Try either of the above tips with softened frozen yogurt. Most brands are safe, but always double-check ingredients as they can change.

Note: Most plain yogurt is safe. Avoid yogurt with crunch toppings and steer toward the all-natural brands with live cultures. These are less apt to be thickened with other things.

LOAD THOSE SPUDS
(CAN YOU TOP THESE BAKED POTATOES?)

- Baked potatoes. Top baked potatoes with vegetables, cheese, and crumbled bacon and heat under the broiler until the cheese melts.
- Chili Potatoes. Spoon leftover chili or soup (see Soup Doctor) over baked spuds.
- Pizza Spuds. Add favorite pizza toppings and heat briefly.
- Kid-Friendly Potato Heads. Let the kids create their own edible potato heads.

NOODLING AROUND

- Noodle Pot. Use this as a geography lesson and combine Asian rice noodles and frozen veggies in gluten-free beef or chicken broth. Add gluten-free soy sauce or hot sauce and slices of meat as desired.
- Pasta Bake. Toss leftover pasta with soup and top with cheese. Brown under the broiler.
- On Top of Ole Smoky: Pasta and Meatballs. Let the kids roll little meatballs and bake them in the oven. Top a bowl full of gluten-free pasta (leftover or freshly cooked) with meatballs, sauce, and cheese. Is there anything more fun than watching spaghetti sauce drizzle down a mound of pasta?

SOUP DOCTOR

- Several companies make soups that are labeled "gluten-free." Doctor them up to make a hearty meal. Let the kids rummage through the refrigerator to find specimens—leftover cubed meat, cold cuts, cheese, rice, cold gluten-free pasta, or frozen vegetables. Add these ingredients to cups of soup and heat in the microwave. Here's another way peer pressure can work in your favor. A kid who hates veggies might eat them this way, *especially* if the other kids are adding them to their soup concoctions.

GF Foods You Can
Serve to Your Fanciest Company

The in-laws are coming for Sunday dinner, or you've invited friends to share a meal. And now, not only are you overwhelmed with the menu, but you have another issue—the GFD. It's time to think outside the box, so put on your apron and start your oven.

My motto is *one for all* when it comes to menus. Start with favorite mainstream recipes and substitute boldly.

- Use gluten-free bread in a favorite stuffing recipe.
- Thicken gravy with rice flour or cornstarch.
- Make a delicious lasagna but use rice noodles (see recipe, page 185).

Have a Quickie (recipe-wise):

- Kebabs (cubes of pork, chicken, or beef) marinated in gluten-free teriyaki sauce
- Pork tenderloin marinated in orange juice, crushed garlic, and wheat-free soy sauce
- Steak with killer gravy (page 184)
- Pulled chicken on corn tortillas (shred gluten-free cooked rotisserie chicken and serve with salsa and guacamole)
- Roasted cod wrapped in prosciutto
- Baked or grilled salmon with mustard, lemon juice, and caper sauce
- Roasted Cornish hens brushed with mustard and honey
- Add your favorite sides: see tips on page 156.
- Keep dessert simple: fresh fruit and sorbet; gluten-free brownies with ice cream.

Baking Basics

Many folks who can cook a meal are overwhelmed when it comes to baking. They didn't bake before they went gluten-free and now the thought of picking up a whisk has them trembling. No worries. Here are a few foolproof ways to guarantee success. The bonus is you get to control the ingredients and avoid the extra fats and sugar often used to keep gluten-free prepared products fresh and tasty.

Stock your pantry with an assortment of gluten-free baking mixes—muffin, cake, pie, bread, and muffins. (If you like a certain brand, buy it by the case at Amazon.com to save money and ensure you won't run out.) Mixes are foolproof and absolve you of the pressure to stock and create flour blends every time you want to bake. (For specific brands, see Resources, page 312.)

Once you become accustomed to the way gluten-free doughs behave and are feeling adventurous, try some from-scratch recipes, such as the ones in this book or from other cookbooks (see Resources, page 305).

Speaking of behavior, gluten-free bread dough does not behave at all like gluten-filled dough. It's a batter constructed from a delicate balance of wet to dry ingredients and way too sticky to knead or handle. The good news is that gluten-free bread dough takes only a fraction of the time to prepare as its gluteny counterpart. The mixture is simply beaten, then transferred to a pan to rise. After about 40 minutes, into the oven it goes, and less than an hour later, it's bread. The texture is a bit more cakey than chewy and the crust is thinner than that of its gluten-filled relatives. But most people find the taste very pleasant. Don't use a dough hook to prepare this dough. The paddle attachment or beaters are more suited to gluten-free baking.

Personalize mixes. Add cinnamon and raisins to bread mixes; frost layer cakes with your favorite buttercream; add chopped fruit or nuts to muffin mixes; and fill piecrust (from a mix or frozen prepared crust) with your favorite pie filling

If you want the most insanely simple piecrust, crush cookies, add 2 to 3 tablespoons of melted butter or coconut butter, and press the mixture into a pie pan. Add your favorite pudding plus sliced fruit or spoon in softened frozen yogurt or ice cream. Top with more crumbs and chill until served. (Use crushed ginger cookies or snickerdoodle cookies as the crust for cheesecake, too.)

When you are feeling adventurous, make my apple pie recipe (page 170). And, when you are ready, try your hand at more advanced baking. For that, you'll need an overview of the many, many flours available to the gluten-free baker.

Flour Power

We are fortunate to have a wide range of gluten-free flours. Many are filled with essential vitamins, minerals, and fiber that add benefits to your diet, too.

Because no single gluten-free flour has all the properties of wheat flour, you'll want to use several to achieve a flour blend that comes close to the Gold Medal you've left behind. It's important to understand the nuances of each flour. Some are high in protein and fiber, but have a distinct flavor; others are neutral but, by themselves, offer a load of empty carbs; still others, starches, have no protein and little nutritional value, but add a lot of lift and texture. Understanding these properties will help you become a better gluten-free baker.

Here are some of the key players. I've coded them to help you identify their function: **N** (neutral), **HPF** (high protein and fiber), **S** (starches), **G** (gums), **TB** (texture builders). You can find many of these at your local health food store; and more and more mainstream groceries are carrying these "alternative" flours and ingredients. Bob's Red Mill makes a wide range of gluten-free ingredients that are available nationally. You can also order ingredients online, stocking up to reduce cost. The flours in each category perform a similar function and are interchangeable. Texture builders are the exception. These are used to add texture, structure or moisture, and are generally not interchangeable and not used in ALL flour blends.

Note: Flours should be stored in airtight containers in the refrigerator or freezer to extend the shelf life.

Neutral (N)

Corn flour (N): This finely ground cornmeal comes in yellow and white. One form of corn flour, masa harina (milled from hominy), is used in making corn tortillas. Corn flour is a good source of vitamins, contains some fiber and protein, and imparts a slightly nutty taste.

Rice flour (N): The workhorse of gluten-free baking, this is available as brown rice (higher in fiber), sweet rice (short grain, with a higher starch content), and white rice. The texture varies depending on how it's milled—fine, medium, or coarse. White rice flour has a bland taste and very little fiber or protein. Brown rice is slightly nutty. Despite the name, sweet rice flour is not sweet.

Sorghum flour (N) & (HPF): Also called milo or jowar flour, the taste is similar to wheat. High in protein and vitamins, it has a slightly sweet taste and works well in most gluten-free recipes.

High Protein and Fiber (HPF)

Amaranth (HPF): Made from the seeds of the broad-leafed amaranth plant, amaranth is very high in protein, fiber, calcium, and iron. Amaranth flour adds structure to gluten-free baked goods and helps them brown more quickly.

Bean flours (HPF): High in protein, fiber, and calcium, the most popular types in gluten-free baking are chickpea (garbanzo), soy flour, and Garfava flour (a blend of garbanzo, fava, and Romano beans). These add elasticity to breads and other baked goods, but have a strong aftertaste, so go light on bean flour. And extra fiber can do a number on delicate digestive systems.

Buckwheat (HPF): Despite its name, buckwheat is not a wheat; it has a strong, robust flavor and is a great source of protein and eight essential amino acids. Use about 20 percent in a flour blend. More can lend a strong flavor.

Flax (HPF) & (TB): Flaxseeds are high in fiber and omega-3 fatty acids. Whole flaxseed is not digestible so buy flaxseed meal (ground flaxseed) or make your own by grinding the seeds in a clean coffee grinder. Store in the refrigerator or freezer. Add 2 to 3 tablespoons of flaxseed meal per recipe for baked goods or sprinkle it on yogurt or cereal for a nutritional boost. A mixture of flaxseed meal and warm water is used as an egg replacer in egg-free baking. (Salba, or chia, is another seed with similar properties and functions.)

Millet (HPF): An ancient food, millet imparts a light beige or yellow color to foods. The flour creates light baked goods and adds a crunch to pizza and bread crust. High in protein and fiber, millet adds structure to gluten-free baked goods. It's not good for use in delicate pastries.

Oat flour (HPF): High in fiber, protein, and nutrition, oats add taste, texture, and structure to cookies, breads, and other baked goods. *Make sure oats are certified gluten-free.*

Quinoa (HPF): Milled from a grain that's native to the Andes Mountains in South America, quinoa ("keen-wah") is actually a seed. It has a delicate, nutty flavor similar to wild rice, and lots of protein, fiber, and vitamins. This superfood is a super flour for gluten-free baking, too.

Teff flour (HPF): Milled from one of the world's smallest grains, teff is high in protein and fiber and a wonderful addition to gluten-free yeast bread blends. It's not recommended for delicate baked goods.

Starches (S)

Arrowroot, cornstarch, potato starch (do not substitute potato flour), and **tapioca starch** (sometimes called tapioca flour) **(S)** are fairly interchangeable in gluten-free blends. These can also be used to thicken gravies, soups, and sauces.

Gums (G)

Agar powder, guar gum, and **xanthan gum (G)** put the "glue" back in gluten-free baking. Use small amounts (see page 165). As you'll see, potato flour can also serve as a binding agent.

Texture Builders (TB)

Almond flour (TB): finely ground almonds. Almonds are a healthy source of manganese and vitamin E, high in protein and low in carbs.

Ground almonds can be added to a blend as one of the flours (use up to 25 percent), or use ¼ to ⅓ cup to add texture to baked goods.

Coconut flour (TB): High in fiber and protein; add a small amount to a baking blend (up to ¼ cup) to add texture. Adding more will mean adding additional liquid, as coconut flour absorbs a lot of moisture.

Flax meal (TB): See Flax.

Potato flour (TB): Made from dehydrated potatoes, this is a fine yellow-white powder that's high in fiber and protein. It's highly absorbent and can be used in place of xanthan gum or guar gum in gluten-free baking. Add no more than 2 to 3 tablespoons per recipe to lend a soft, chewy mouthfeel to baked goods. Too much can create a gummy texture. Don't confuse potato flour with potato starch, which contains no protein and is used in much larger quantities in a recipe.

Make a Blend

A good blend is a balance of neutral flour, high-protein flour, starch, and a small amount of a gum. Start with this ratio, selecting one type of flour from each category.

2 CUPS NEUTRAL FLOUR
- White or brown rice
- Corn
- Sorghum (fits both categories)

1 CUP HIGH-PROTEIN/HIGH-FIBER FLOUR
- Amaranth
- Chickpea
- Millet
- Oat
- Quinoa
- Sorghum
- Teff

2 CUPS STARCH

- Arrowroot
- Cornstarch
- Potato starch
- Tapioca starch

GUMS
(ADD ACCORDING TO THE FORMULA BELOW)

- Agar powder
- Guar gum
- Xanthan gum

Add gums as follows:

- For cookies: ½ teaspoon gum per 1 cup of blend
- For cakes and cupcakes: ¾ teaspoon per 1 cup of blend
- For yeast breads: 1 teaspoon per 1 cup of blend
- For pizza and piecrust: 1½ teaspoons per 1 cup of blend

TEXTURE BUILDERS
(NOT PART OF A BASIC BLEND BUT OFTEN
USED TO ADD TEXTURE AS DESCRIBED ABOVE)

- Almond flour
- Coconut flour
- Flax meal
- Potato flour (not starch)

Try switching around the neutral and protein flour so you have two cups of protein flour and one cup of neutral flour when making breads or pizza. Try adding ½ cup of almond flour or ¼ cup flax meal for texture in quick breads, cookies, and muffins. Use a blend of sorghum flour, rice flour, and cornstarch for layer cakes. I've made up sample blends here:

All-Purpose Flour Blend

Good for cookies, cakes, scones, biscotti, and as a 1:1 replacement for regular flour in your favorite family recipes.

Add the correct amount of gum according to the kind of recipe you are making. Try adding 2 to 3 tablespoons of almond flour or flax meal to this blend to boost texture.

2 cups white rice flour
1 cup sorghum
1 cup potato starch (not potato flour) or cornstarch
1 cup tapioca starch

High-Protein Flour Blend

Good for yeast breads, pizza, piecrust, and more. Use as a 1:1 replacement for whole wheat flour.

Add the correct amount of gum according to the kind of recipe you are making. Try adding 2 to 3 tablespoons of flax meal or potato flour to this blend to boost texture.

1 cup sorghum or chickpea flour
1 cup millet, sorghum, or amaranth flour
1 cup brown or white rice flour
1 cup potato starch (not potato flour) or cornstarch
1 cup tapioca starch

Now you have a blend that's ready to use as a cup-for-cup replacement for regular flour or whole wheat flour in your favorite recipes. Switch out the flours as you experiment. Once you have a blend you like, multiply by two or five or ten to make a large quantity that can be ready anytime you want to bake. Don't add the gum until you know what recipe you are making. If time is short, replace your blend with a commercial gluten-free blend. If the mix contains gum and salt, do not add these again.

Storing Your Baked Goods

Who wants to make an entire batch of cookies, brownies, or cupcakes for one person? Here's where a freezer comes in handy. Wrap leftovers in serving-size portions and freeze. (Slice breads before wrapping for the freezer.) These can be a godsend when you need a quick snack or treat, when your child needs a cupcake for a birthday party, or when soccer practice is moments away and you have nothing to feed your kid. To revive your frozen baked goods, wrap a single serving in a paper towel and microwave for 30 to 45 seconds to thaw. Warm in a 350°F oven until heated through or toast breads. Thaw cookies and brownies at room temperature.

Safe Substitutions

You may have additional food sensitivities besides gluten. If a recipe includes one of those ingredients, there's no need to write it off. Just bake around it by replacing ingredients with foods you can have.

Once you create a list of safe substitutions, foods you can have, it's easy to come up with good alternatives for every recipe. Here are a few examples.

Dairy

Replace cow's milk with an equal amount of:

> Almond milk
> Coconut milk
> Fruit juice (orange or apple)
> Hemp milk
> Soy milk

Use unsweetened varieties unless specified. Flavored, sweetened versions of these can add too much sweetener to recipes that already call for sugar.

Butter

Replace with an equal amount of:

Coconut oil
Fleischmann's Unsalted Margarine (contains whey)
Earth Balance Natural Shortening Sticks (earthbalancenatural.com)
Earth Balance Vegan Buttery Sticks (earthbalancenatural.com)
Spectrum Organic Shortening (spectrumorganics.com)
Smart Balance Buttery Spread (contains whey)

Sour Cream or Yogurt

Replace with an equal amount of:

Almond yogurt
Coconut yogurt
Rice yogurt
Soy yogurt

Eggs

Replace with the following:

Use this formula to replace one large egg: 1 tablespoon of flax meal or
chia seeds mixed with 3 tablespoons of hot water. Let stand until
thick (about 5 minutes). Add when the recipe calls for eggs.
Ener-G egg replacer (prepare according to the package directions)

Must-Haves for a Well-Equipped Gluten-free Baker

- Vegetable cooking spray (check labels as some contain flour)
- Ice-cream scoops of all sizes (easy way to transfer dough and batter
  and makes perfect shapes)

- Plastic wrap (a workhorse in the kitchen; creates a barrier between fingers and sticky gluten-free dough; great for smoothing tops of breads, and spreading pizza and piecrust)
- Instant-read thermometer (to check the internal temperature of breads and rolls for doneness)
- Proofer (an appliance that creates a warm, draft-free environment so yeast doughs can rise to the max)

Bread Machine

A bread machine is a must if you like to make homemade gluten-free bread. Select a machine that comes with a gluten-free cycle or one that can be programmed to use only one knead and rise cycle. Additional knead and rise cycles are not necessary for gluten-free breads and may even prevent your loaf from rising properly. (See a list of GFF bread machines in Resources, page 315.)

Heavy-Duty Mixer

Gluten-free dough is much heavier than gluten-filled dough. Invest in a heavy-duty stand mixer, such as one made by KitchenAid, Cuisinart, or Breville. If budget or space is an issue, a heavy-duty handheld mixer with a 225- or 250-watt motor can be purchased from one of these companies. Your gluten-free baking will thank you.

Recipes: 15 Favorite Foods You Never Thought You'd Eat Again and How to Make Them

For many of us, a diagnosis brings relief—and a pretty big sadness that we can no longer have some of our favorite foods again (Grandma's apple pie recipe? Forget it. The chicken and dumplings you had on every major birthday? Nope). Following are fifteen recipes for some basic favorites—both savory and sweet—proving that you may give up gluten, but you won't be giving up flavor, texture, or deliciousness.

Apple Pie with Flaky Piecrust
Banana Bread
Buttermilk Biscuits
Birthday Cake
Chicken and Parsley Dumplings
Chicken Parmesan
Chocolate Chip Cookies
Doughnut Rounds
French Bread Baguettes
Great Gravy: A Master Recipe
Lasagna with Beef and Spinach
Oven-Fried Chicken
Pizza with Cheese and Tomatoes
Sandwich Bread
Soft Pretzels

Apple Pie with Flaky Piecrust

Makes one 9-inch pie

Into every life a little pie must land. And this one will land softly and lightly. Despite the absence of gluten, the crust is flaky and delicate and it tastes like it came right out of Grandma's kitchen. The dough is not prone to tear, but if it does, simply pat it back into place. If you're craving something other than apple, just use your favorite gluten-free filling and bake according to the pie filling recipe's instructions, or use the one I've provided here.

½ cup amaranth flour
½ cup white rice flour
6 tablespoons cornstarch or potato starch (not potato flour)
¼ cup tapioca starch
1 tablespoon potato flour (not potato starch)
1 teaspoon xanthan gum
¼ teaspoon salt

2 to 3 teaspoons sugar
½ teaspoon baking powder
½ teaspoon ground cinnamon
4 tablespoons cold butter or dairy-free butter replacement
4 tablespoons organic shortening
1 teaspoon cider vinegar
2 tablespoons unsweetened applesauce
1 large egg, or 2 tablespoons additional unsweetened applesauce
1 large egg, lightly beaten, for brushing

▶ In the bowl of a food processor fitted with the knife blade, combine the dry ingredients (including the xanthan gum). Cut the butter and shortening into pieces. Sprinkle over the dry ingredients. Pulse several times until the pieces are the size of large peas.

▶ In a separate bowl, combine the vinegar, the 2 tablespoons of applesauce, and one egg (or the additional applesauce). Add to the flour mixture and process just to combine. Carefully gather the dough into a ball. (Watch your fingers as the steel knife is very sharp.) Wrap in plastic wrap and chill for 1 hour. If refrigerated longer, let stand at room temperature until pliable.

▶ Make the apple filling that follows, or use your favorite recipe.

▶ Preheat the oven to 425°F. Lightly oil a 9-inch pie pan. Reserve about one quarter of the dough. Place the remaining dough between two layers of plastic wrap and press it down with heel of your hand. Start from the middle and gently roll out uniformly in all directions to form a 9½-inch circle. Rotate the dough in one-quarter turns to help even out the crust to about an ⅛-inch thickness throughout.

▶ Carefully peel off the top layer of plastic wrap. Turn the crust into the pan, slowly peeling off the backing. Press the crust into the pan. Trim off any excess dough, leaving a little overhanging beyond the lip, and set aside. (Add the scraps to the reserved dough.) Crimp the edges of the piecrust. Roll out the reserved dough to a long rectangle of ⅛-inch thickness. Cut into eight strips.

▶ Prick the bottom of the crust and brush with beaten egg. Add the apple mixture, mounding it slightly in the center.

▶ Crisscross the top with the strips of dough to create a lattice effect. Brush the strips with beaten egg and set the pie in the preheated oven. Bake for 15 minutes. Lower the heat to 350°F. Continue baking for 35 to 45 minutes, until the apples are soft and the filling bubbles. If the crust begins to brown before the filling is cooked, tent the crust with aluminum foil.

APPLE PIE FILLING

6 Macoun or other apples, peeled and thinly sliced
½ cup sugar
2 tablespoons cornstarch
¼ teaspoon salt
1 teaspoon ground cinnamon
¼ teaspoon ground nutmeg
¼ teaspoon ground allspice
2 teaspoons freshly squeezed lemon juice
3 tablespoons cold unsalted butter, cut into small pieces

▶ Toss the apples with the remaining ingredients. Fill the piecrust and bake according to instructions above.

Banana Bread

Yields 12 to 14 slices

Everyone needs an easy gluten-free quick bread in his or her repertoire. Delicious and versatile, this will become your go-to quick bread. You can keep it simple or dress this up by adding toasted coarsely chopped pecans, chocolate chips, or coconut. Swap the bananas for the same amount of pumpkin or sweet potato puree for another treat. For the best flavor, use very ripe bananas, the kind you'd be tempted to throw away. If yours are not overly ripe, add ½ to 1 teaspoon of banana extract to perk up the flavor.

¾ cup white rice flour
½ cup sorghum flour
½ cup cornstarch or tapioca starch
¼ cup potato starch (not potato flour)
2 teaspoons xanthan gum
1½ teaspoons baking powder
½ teaspoon baking soda
½ teaspoon salt
1 teaspoon ground cinnamon
¼ teaspoon ground nutmeg
½ cup granulated sugar

½ cup packed light brown sugar
½ cup (1 stick) cold unsalted butter, cut into small pieces
1⅓ cups very ripe mashed bananas (about 3 large bananas)
1 teaspoon pure vanilla extract
2 large eggs

▸ Preheat the oven to 350°F. Lightly grease a 9 x 5-inch loaf pan.

▸ In a large mixing bowl, whisk together the rice flour, sorghum flour, cornstarch, potato starch, xanthan gum, baking powder, baking soda, salt, cinnamon, and nutmeg. Set aside.

▸ In the bowl of a food processor fitted with the knife blade, place the two sugars and the butter. Pulse until the mixture is crumbly, about 30 seconds. Add the bananas and vanilla, and pulse to combine. Add the eggs. Pulse until smooth.

▸ Add the dry ingredients and pulse for about 30 seconds, or until the mixture is thick and smooth.

▸ Transfer to the prepared loaf pan. Set in the middle of the preheated oven and bake for 45 to 50 minutes. Remove from the oven, allow to set in the pan for 10 minutes, then turn out onto a wire rack to cool completely.

▸ Wrapped in plastic wrap, this freezes well and will keep for 3 to 6 months.

Birthday Cake

Makes two 8- or 9-inch layers or 36 cupcakes

No reason to go without birthday cake just because you are gluten-free. This light, airy layer cake has "celebration" written all over it. Add your favorite icing and decorations and let everyone enjoy. Turn this batter into cupcakes, too. Frost and decorate as many as you need and freeze the rest for another celebration.

1½ cups white rice flour, plus extra to coat pans
¾ cup sorghum flour
¾ cup cornstarch or potato starch (not potato flour)
¼ cup tapioca starch

3 teaspoons baking powder
2 teaspoons xanthan gum
¾ teaspoon salt
¾ cup (1½ sticks) unsalted butter, at room temperature
2 cups sugar
2 teaspoons vanilla extract
4 large eggs, at room temperature
1¼ cups milk, at room temperature

▶ Preheat the oven to 375°F. Lightly grease two 8- or 9-inch round cake pans that are at least 2 inches deep. Coat with rice flour. Shake out the excess flour. Set aside. (Or line three 12-cup muffin tins with cupcake papers.)

▶ In a medium-size mixing bowl, whisk together the rice flour, sorghum flour, cornstarch, tapioca starch, baking powder, xanthan gum, and salt. Set aside.

▶ In a large bowl, beat the butter, sugar, and vanilla until smooth.

▶ Add the eggs one at a time, beating at medium speed just until they're incorporated and scraping the bottom of the bowl after each addition.

▶ Add the flour mixture alternately with the milk, mixing at low speed to incorporate. Scrape the sides of the bowl after each addition. Begin and end with the flour mixture. Once the last of the flour mixture is added, mix briefly, just until smooth.

▶ Divide the batter between the pans. Weigh out the batter if you want the layers to be exactly even. Smooth the top of each pan. (Or half-fill each muffin cup with batter.)

▶ Bake the cakes for 28 to 30 minutes for 8-inch cakes, 26 to 28 minutes for 9-inch cakes (18 to 20 minutes for cupcakes), until evenly browned and a cake tester inserted into the center of one layer (or cupcake) comes out clean.

▶ Remove from the oven, and allow to cool in the pan for 10 minutes. Run a spatula around the edges to loosen, and turn onto a rack to cool completely before frosting. Or wrap well and freeze 3 to 6 months.

Tip: The cakes can be cut through the center and frosted to create a four-layer cake.

Buttermilk Biscuits

Makes ten 2½-inch biscuits (more if a smaller biscuit cutter is used)

Once I was diagnosed, I feared I'd never again be able to have hot biscuits straight from the oven, the kind my mother made when I was a kid. But these light, fluffy, buttery biscuits take me back to that time when I could enjoy this treat with the rest of the family.

A couple of tips:

Cornstarch helps produce a more tender biscuit. However, if you can't have corn products, you can substitute tapioca starch with good results.

To get the maximum lift from these biscuits, use a sharp biscuit cutter and do not twist the cutter as you remove it from the dough. If you don't have a round biscuit cutter, pat the dough into a rectangle and cut into squares. They'll still taste delicious.

1 cup white or brown rice flour
¾ cup sorghum flour
⅓ cup cornstarch or tapioca starch
1 tablespoon baking powder
2 teaspoons sugar
¾ teaspoon xanthan gum
½ teaspoon salt
½ teaspoon baking soda
4 tablespoons unsalted cold butter or dairy-free alternative
3 tablespoons organic vegetable shortening
¾ cup buttermilk
1 tablespoon melted butter, to brush the tops of the biscuits

- ▶ Preheat the oven to 425°F. Line a baking sheet with parchment paper. Set aside.

- ▶ In the bowl of a food processor fitted with the knife blade, pulse the rice flour, sorghum flour, cornstarch, baking powder, sugar, xanthan gum, salt, and baking soda.

- ▶ Cut the butter and shortening into small pieces. Scatter the pieces of butter and shortening over the top of the flour mixture. Pulse in 3-second pulses until the mixture is crumbly, about 30 seconds. Add the buttermilk and process until smooth, about 30 seconds.

▶ Spread a sheet of plastic wrap or parchment paper on the counter. Turn out the dough onto the plastic sheet. Knead and pat into a ½- to ¾-inch-thick circle. Use a 2¼-inch round biscuit cutter to cut as many biscuits as possible from the dough. Set them on the prepared baking sheet.

▶ Gather the dough scraps and pat into another circle of the same thickness and cut out as many biscuits as possible. Repeat until all the dough is used.

▶ Brush the tops with melted butter and bake for 12 to 15 minutes, or until the tops are golden brown. Remove from the oven and allow to cool slightly. Serve immediately.

▶ The biscuits can be frozen and reheated for 5 minutes at 350°F before serving. However, these are best straight from the oven, just like Mom served them.

Variation: Add 1¼ cups of shredded Cheddar cheese with the buttermilk for cheesy biscuits.

Chicken Parmesan

Serves 4

This GF Chicken Parmesan is a great do-ahead dish and kid-friendly, too. If you are avoiding dairy, replace the cheese with dairy-free substitutes or omit.

4 boneless, skinless chicken breast cutlets
   (about 1¼ pounds)
1 (24- to 26-ounce jar) good-quality chunky-style marinara sauce,
   more for pasta
2 cloves garlic, minced
3 teaspoons chopped fresh basil
3 large eggs
½ cup white rice flour
1 teaspoon dried Italian seasoning
Salt and freshly ground black pepper

2 cups gluten-free bread crumbs
  (see Resources for brands, page 312)
2 to 4 tablespoons extra-virgin olive oil,
  or more as needed
8 slices provolone cheese
½ cup shredded Parmesan cheese, or more if desired
1 (12-ounce) package gluten-free spaghetti

- ▸ Preheat the oven to 375°F. Lightly oil a 9 x 13-inch Pyrex baking dish. Set aside. Start heating a large pot of salted water so it will be boiling when you are ready to make the spaghetti.

- ▸ Cut the chicken cutlets into serving-size portions. In a medium-size saucepan, heat the marinara sauce with the garlic. When it begins to steam, add the basil and remove from the heat. Set aside.

- ▸ Beat the eggs in a shallow bowl. In another shallow bowl, place the rice flour, Italian seasoning, and salt and pepper. Whisk with a fork to combine. Place the bread crumbs in another bowl.

- ▸ Line a cookie sheet with aluminum foil or parchment paper. Dip a chicken cutlet in the beaten egg. Then dip it in the flour mixture until evenly coated. Dip the cutlet back in the egg and then into the bread crumbs, pressing the crumbs into both sides. Set on the lined cookie sheet. Repeat with each cutlet.

- ▸ Heat a large skillet over medium-high heat. Pour in 2 tablespoons of olive oil and heat until it begins to shimmer. Add two or three cutlets at a time and cook for about 3 minutes on each side. Transfer to the prepared baking dish and repeat until all the cutlets are browned. Add more oil as needed.

- ▸ Pour the warm sauce over the chicken. Top with provolone cheese and sprinkle Parmesan cheese over the top.

- ▸ Bake for 15 minutes, or until the cheese is bubbly and the chicken is no longer pink in the center.

- ▸ While the chicken is baking, cook the spaghetti according to the package directions. Serve with the chicken. Pass additional sauce and cheese, if desired.

- ▸ This dish (without the spaghetti) can be made ahead and stored in the refrigerator for 24 hours. Reheat covered in a 325°F oven for 15 minutes.

Chicken and Parsley Dumplings

Serves 4 to 6

This is one of the most frequently asked-for recipes when people are new to the gluten-free diet. How ironic that the gluten-filled version of this wholesome comfort food is one that many of us sought out when we were feeling poorly before diagnosis. This rendition is tummy-trouble-free and reheats well.

CHICKEN AND VEGETABLES

1 tablespoon olive oil
1 medium-size onion, roughly chopped
2 cloves garlic, minced
¼ cup dry sherry or vermouth (optional)
1 quart gluten-free chicken broth, or more as needed
1 pound boneless, skinless chicken breast, or 3 cups cubed gluten-free
    precooked rotisserie chicken (see note about rotisserie chicken)
1 teaspoon dried thyme
6 sprigs of fresh flat-leaf parsley
Salt and freshly ground black pepper
1 large potato, peeled and cubed
1 (12-ounce) package frozen mixed vegetables (about 2½ cups)

PARSLEY DUMPLINGS

Makes about 18 dumplings

¾ cup white or brown rice flour
¾ cup potato starch (not potato flour)
½ cup sorghum flour
1 teaspoon xanthan gum
3 teaspoons baking powder
¾ teaspoon salt
¼ cup chopped flat-leaf parsley
1 tablespoon dehydrated chives
¾ cup plus 2 tablespoons milk of choice
2 tablespoons butter, melted
1 large egg, beaten

▶ Prepare the chicken and vegetables: In a large pot with a tightly fitting lid, combine the olive oil, onion, and garlic. Sauté until the onion is translucent. Add the sherry and simmer until the liquid is reduced by half. Add the chicken broth and bring the liquid to a gentle simmer. Add the chicken breasts, thyme, parsley, and salt and pepper to taste. Poach covered for 5 minutes. Using a slotted spoon, remove the breasts and allow to cool. Skim any foam off the surface of the liquid.

▶ Return the pot of chicken broth to medium-high heat. Add the potatoes. Cover and simmer until just fork tender (about 10 minutes), while making the dumplings.

▶ Make the dumpling batter: Whisk together the rice flour, potato starch, sorghum flour, xanthan gum, baking powder, and salt in a medium-size bowl. Add the parsley and chives and mix well. Add the milk, melted butter, and egg to the dry ingredients. Gently mix with a wooden spoon or a fork until the mixture is moist and comes together. Do not overmix or the dumplings will be too dense.

▶ Cube the chicken and return to the pot along with the frozen vegetables. Add additional broth if the mixture is too thick or the liquid has cooked down too much. Return to a simmer.

▶ Drop the dumpling batter by heaping tablespoonfuls into the simmering stew, to cover the surface of the stew. (Note that the dumplings will double in size as they cook.) Cover and simmer until the dumplings are cooked through, about 15 minutes. Do not uncover and peek while the dumplings are cooking. For the dumplings to be light and fluffy, they must steam, not boil.

▶ If after 15 minutes they are still not cooked through (use a toothpick or skewer to test), cover the pan again and cook for another 5 minutes.

▶ Ladle portions of meat, sauce, vegetables, and dumplings into soup plates and serve. Note that the stew will continue to thicken as it sits.

▶ Keep refrigerated and enjoy within 3 days.

Note: If rotisserie chicken is used, there's no need to poach the chicken. Simply cube and add the chicken just before adding the dumpling mixture. Add the thyme, parsley, and salt and pepper to the chicken broth when adding the potatoes.

Chocolate Chip (a.k.a. Toll House) Cookies

Makes 50 to 55 (3-inch) cookies

While growing up, I made hundreds of batches of these famous cookies. I'm sure you did, too. When I gave up gluten, I thought I'd be missing out on these babies, too. But by using a blend of gluten-free flours that includes cornstarch and sorghum, I was able to create a version that will have everyone fooled.

1 cup white or brown rice flour
½ cup sorghum flour
½ cup cornstarch or tapioca starch
¼ cup potato starch (not potato flour)
1 teaspoon xanthan gum
1 teaspoon baking soda
8 ounces (2 sticks) unsalted butter or dairy-free buttery sticks,
    at room temperature (see note)
¾ teaspoon salt
2 teaspoons pure vanilla extract
¾ cup granulated sugar
¾ cup firmly packed light brown sugar
2 large eggs
2 cups gluten-free semisweet chocolate chips (see note)

- ▶ Line four cookie sheets with parchment paper.
- ▶ In a medium-size mixing bowl, whisk together the rice flour, sorghum flour, cornstarch, potato starch, xanthan gum, and baking soda. Set aside.
- ▶ In a large mixing bowl, cream the butter until fluffy. Add the salt and vanilla and beat. Add the two sugars. Beat well until the mixture is smooth. Add the eggs and beat. Add half of the flour mixture at a time, beating after each addition. Fold in the chocolate chips.
- ▶ Refrigerate the dough for 1 hour. (If you are pressed for time, omit this step; if you omit, preheat the oven before step one of the directions.) Preheat the oven to 375°F.
- ▶ Drop the cookie dough by heaping teaspoonfuls about 2 inches apart onto the prepared cookie sheets. Bake for 12 to 14 minutes, or until the tops are slightly browned. Remove from the oven and allow to cool

completely before removing from the cookie sheets. While these are bak-ing and cooling, drop the remaining dough onto the other pans. If your kitchen is very warm, keep these chilled until you are ready to bake.

▶ These freeze well. The dough can be scooped into balls and frozen, then stored in a resealable plastic bag to bake later.

Notes: Nondairy buttery sticks will not spread as much as butter. Flat-ten the balls of dough slightly on the cookie sheets before baking.

If you are avoiding dairy, dairy-free chocolate chips are available from EnjoyLifeFoods.com.

Doughnut Rounds (a.k.a. Munchkins)

Makes 36 to 40 doughnut rounds

Perhaps you thought it was impossible to have great doughnuts when you went gluten-free. But rest assured, it's not true. You'll agree when you bite into these light and cakey little gems. The almond flour and powdered whey add texture and protein to this recipe.

You'll need a candy thermometer to make these.

4 tablespoons unsalted butter
2 tablespoons honey
½ cup white rice flour
6 tablespoons sorghum flour
¼ cup plus 1 tablespoon cornstarch or potato starch
   (not potato flour)
3 tablespoons tapioca starch
3 tablespoons whey powder or powdered skim milk
3 tablespoons almond flour
2 tablespoons sugar
2 teaspoons xanthan gum
¼ teaspoon salt
1½ teaspoons rapid-rise yeast
1 large egg plus 1 large egg yolk
1 teaspoon lemon zest (optional)
3 to 4 cups canola or grapeseed oil, for frying

COATING

3 tablespoons granulated sugar plus 2 teaspoons ground cinnamon
(or just use confectioners' sugar without any cinnamon)

▶ Heat ½ cup of water until very warm but not boiling. Add the butter and
honey and stir until melted. Set aside and allow to cool to about 100°F.

▶ In the bowl of a stand mixer fitted with the paddle attachment (or a
large mixing bowl), beat the rice flour, sorghum flour, cornstarch, tapioca starch, whey powder, almond flour, sugar, xanthan gum, and salt
until well combined. Add the yeast and beat to combine. Add the butter
mixture and beat just to moisten. Add the egg, egg yolk, and the lemon
zest, if using, and beat until smooth and the dough begins to pull away
from the sides of the bowl. Remove the bowl from the mixer. With oiled
fingers, pat the dough into a smooth ball. Cover with a sheet of plastic
wrap and set in a warm, draft-free area until the dough has doubled in
size (about 1 hour).

▶ Line two cookie sheets with parchment paper and spray with vegetable spray. Using a 1-inch scoop, scoop out portions of dough and drop
them on the parchment paper. Gently roll each portion on the paper to
create a smooth ball. Let the dough rest for 20 to 30 minutes, or until
the balls have risen slightly.

▶ Combine the sugar and cinnamon on a medium-size plate. Line a large
plate with paper towels. Line another cookie sheet with parchment
paper.

▶ In a deep skillet or saucepan, heat the oil until it registers about 360°F
on a candy thermometer. Add four or five balls of dough at a time, turning so they brown evenly. They will cook very quickly. Transfer to the
paper towel–lined plate.

▶ Toss with the cinnamon-sugar mixture to coat. Serve warm. These can
be stored at room temperature for 1 to 2 days, but don't freeze them.

Note: Because these brown quickly, cut one open to make sure it's
cooked through. If not, place the doughnuts on a baking sheet and bake
in a preheated 350°F oven for 3 minutes before coating in sugar. Do not
overbake these. The centers should not be cakey.

French Bread Baguettes

Makes 2 baguettes

Chewy texture and crusty exterior were hardly descriptions of gluten-free bread when I started this journey. My essay "The Big Chew: A History of Bread" (page 132) chronicles the many iterations of bread that I encountered and endured in the early gluten-free days, as well as the new, improved breads of late. However, this recipe has them all beat. It is chewy, with a great crust and wonderful flavor. If you didn't know better, you'd say you were eating *real* French bread. The secret is psyllium husk, the new darling of the gluten-free baking world. You may recall psyllium is the basis of colon cleansers. Don't let that freak you out. When psyllium combines with liquid, it produces a gelatinous mixture that is great for bread baking. Form this into baguettes or boules (round loaves) or one of each.

1 cup millet flour
1 cup sorghum flour
1 cup sweet rice flour
½ cup cornmeal
1½ teaspoons salt
⅓ cup whole psyllium husk
¼ cup flax meal
2½ cups warm water (105° to 110°F)
4 teaspoons active dry yeast
2½ tablespoons honey
2½ tablespoons olive oil, plus more to brush the tops of the dough

▸ In a medium-size bowl, combine the millet flour, sorghum flour, ¾ cup of the sweet rice flour, and the cornmeal and salt. Set aside. Measure the psyllium husk and flax meal into a small bowl. Set aside.

▸ To the warm water, add the yeast and honey. Stir to combine and let sit until the yeast begins to bubble.

▸ Add the psyllium husk mixture to the yeast mixture and mix well. Let sit for about 5 minutes, or until the mixture thickens. Add 2 tablespoons of the olive oil and mix. Add this mixture to the dry ingredients. Beat for 2 to 3 minutes, or until well combined.

- In a large bowl, add the remaining ¼ cup of sweet rice flour. Turn out the dough into the bowl and knead until the flour mixture is fully incorporated.

- Drizzle the remaining 1½ teaspoons olive oil down the inside of the bowl (not on top of the dough) and turn the dough to coat with the oil. Cover with plastic wrap and set in a warm area for 30 to 40 minutes, or until doubled in size.

- Place a baking stone on the lowest rack of the oven or set a baking rack on the lowest rack in the oven. Preheat the oven to 400°F. Lightly oil a double- or triple-channel baguette pan. (You'll use only two channels.)

- While the oven is preheating, cut the dough in half and roll each piece into a baguette about 14 inches in length. Use oiled plastic wrap to form the loaves, then transfer each to a channel of the pan, using the plastic wrap. Slide the plastic wrap out from under the baguette as you roll it into the pan. Repeat with the remaining dough. Cover with plastic wrap and let rise while the oven preheats (about 20 minutes).

- Brush the tops of the baguettes with olive oil. Set the pan on the stone and bake for 30 to 35 minutes. Turn off the oven. Remove the pan and set a piece of parchment paper on the baking stone. Turn the baguettes onto the stone and let the bread sit in the oven while the oven cools. This puts a terrific crust on the bread.

- Let cool completely before slicing, or the center will be gummy.

- This bread will keep on the counter for up to 3 days and freezes well. (Slice before freezing.)

Variations: Form half of the dough into a baguette and the other half into a round loaf. Let both rise while the oven preheats. Bake the round loaf on a sheet of parchment set directly on the baking stone or on a baking sheet. Or form the dough into one large, round boule loaf and bake for 40 to 45 minutes.

Great Gravy: A Master Recipe

Makes 2 cups

Many people come from the school of flour-thickened gravy and seem intimidated by making gluten-free gravy. Here's an easy recipe that has many variations. Change it to fit each dish: vary the acid (lemon or orange juice, wine, or sherry); add vegetable, beef, or chicken broth; and fold in vegetables of choice (mushrooms, carrots, or roasted onions). Sometimes I like to "finish" my gravy with a splash of cream, a dollop of sour cream, a tablespoon of tomato paste, or a swirl of butter for enrichment. If juices collect in the roasting pan or after the meat or poultry has been cut, strain and add those, too. You decide.

3 tablespoons unsalted butter or olive oil
2 shallots or 1 small onion, minced
⅓ cup dry sherry or white wine
2 cups gluten-free chicken, beef, or vegetable broth
2 tablespoons cornstarch or arrowroot powder
3 tablespoons orange juice or additional broth
Salt and freshly ground black pepper
2 tablespoons half-and-half
1 cup sliced mushrooms, or ½ cup shredded carrot,
   sautéed in butter to soften

▶ In a medium-size saucepan, heat the butter until foamy. Add the shallots and sauté until soft, but do not allow to brown. Add the sherry and simmer until reduced by half. Add the broth and simmer until reduced to 1½ cups. Strain out the shallots, if desired. Add the pan juices here if you have them.

▶ Combine the cornstarch and orange juice and stir well. Bring the gravy mixture to a simmer and stir in the cornstarch mixture. Stir until thickened. Adjust the seasonings. Add the half-and-half and sautéed vegetables, if using. If you like thicker gravy, add up to 2 tablespoons of additional cornstarch mixed with enough liquid to create a smooth mixture.

▶ Serve hot.

▶ The gravy will keep for 2 to 3 days in the refrigerator. It does not freeze well.

Lasagna with Beef and Spinach

Serves 8 to 10

A good recipe for lasagna is essential in any gluten-free kitchen. This one is colorful and hearty and will fool everyone into thinking it's a regular, gluten-filled masterpiece. You can replace the ground beef with ground turkey or crumbled sausage, or combine coarsely chopped veggies and meat, or just use veggies. Lasagna is a very forgiving dish that's delicious with any number of combos. The fact that it is also gluten-free can be your secret. The trick is to undercook the noodles so they do not break apart while assembling and baking this dish.

15 brown rice or corn lasagna noodles
1 (8-ounce) bag baby spinach
2 tablespoons olive oil
1 large shallot, minced
2 cloves garlic, minced
1½ pounds ground beef
Salt and freshly ground black pepper
2 pounds part-skim ricotta cheese or dairy-free ricotta replacement
4 large eggs
2 tablespoons dried parsley, or 4 tablespoons chopped fresh
4 cups good-quality gluten-free marinara sauce
2 cups low-fat mozzarella cheese, shredded, or dairy-free cheese
1 cup grated Parmesan, Romano, or dairy-free cheese

▸ In a large pot, bring 6 quarts of water to a boil. Stir in 1 teaspoon of salt. Add the pasta and cook until softened but not fully cooked, about 6 minutes. Rinse with cold water and drain. Lay the noodles flat on foil-lined baking sheet to cool.

▸ Preheat the oven to 375°F.

▸ In a large skillet, sauté the spinach in 1 tablespoon of the olive oil just until wilted. Remove from the pan and transfer to a plate to cool. Add the remaining 1 tablespoon of oil and sauté the minced shallot for 3 minutes. Add the garlic and ground beef and sauté just until the beef is browned and no pink remains. Add salt and pepper, to taste.

▸ In a small bowl, combine the ricotta cheese, eggs, and parsley. Add the spinach and mix well.

▸ Spread a small amount of marinara sauce in the bottom of a 2-inch deep, 9 x 13-inch pan. Arrange four lasagna noodles lengthwise over the sauce and one perpendicular to the other four, overlapping the edges. Spread half of the ricotta mixture over the pasta. Arrange half of the beef over the ricotta. Sprinkle with ¾ cup of the mozzarella and ½ cup of the Parmesan. Top with another layer of lasagna noodles, followed by half of the remaining marinara sauce. Layer with the remaining ricotta mixture, beef, and ¾ cup of mozzarella. Top with the remaining lasagna noodles. Spoon the remaining marinara sauce over the pasta.

- Cover the lasagna loosely with oiled aluminum foil. Set on a baking sheet and bake for 30 minutes. Remove the foil and top with the remaining mozzarella and Parmesan cheese. Bake for 30 minutes, or until hot and bubbly. Remove from the oven and let stand for 10 minutes before serving, or serve at room temperature.

- Leftovers can be frozen for up to 3 months. Reheat thawed lasagna briefly in the microwave or covered and warmed in a 350°F oven for 15 minutes, or until warmed through.

Oven-Fried Chicken

Serves 3 to 4

Gluten-free or not, we could all take it easy on the fried foods. But I've found an easy way to create crispy foods by baking them at a high temperature. While this baked-not-fried chicken might sound like an oxymoron, it has all the appeal without the extra oil. If you prefer the real deal, you can fry this chicken. See my note below.

> 4 boneless, skinless chicken breast halves (about 1.4 pounds)
> 2 cups low-fat buttermilk
> ½ teaspoon chipotle chili powder
> 1½ cups all-purpose gluten-free flour blend or rice flour
> ½ cup corn flour
> 2 tablespoons plus 2 teaspoons seasoned salt
> 3 teaspoons smoky paprika
> Freshly ground black pepper
> 1½ cups gluten-free bread crumbs
> ½ teaspoon dried thyme
> 2 large eggs
> 2 tablespoons olive oil

- Cut the chicken breasts in half through the thickness to yield eight cutlets.

- In a medium-size bowl, combine the buttermilk and chipotle chili powder. Add the chicken and stir to coat. Let stand, refrigerated, for 30 to 60 minutes.

- In a plate, whisk together the flour mixture, corn flour, 2 tablespoons of the seasoned salt, and the paprika and black pepper.

▸ In a second plate, whisk together the bread crumbs, the remaining 2 teaspoons of seasoned salt, and the thyme.

▸ In a shallow bowl, mix the eggs with 2 tablespoons of water.

▸ Preheat the oven to 400°F. Line a baking sheet with parchment paper or aluminum foil and coat with olive oil.

▸ Remove the chicken from the buttermilk. Shake the excess buttermilk off the chicken pieces. Dredge in the flour mixture to completely coat each piece. Dip in the egg mixture. Then press into the bread crumb mixture to coat on both sides. Set on the prepared baking sheet.

▸ Bake for 15 minutes. Turn and bake for about 10 minutes more, depending on the thickness of the chicken.

Note: To fry the chicken, omit the egg and bread crumb mixtures and simply coat with the flour mixture. Heat ½ cup of oil in a 2- to 3-inch deep, 12-inch skillet and fry on both sides until the internal temperature of the chicken reaches 165°F. Drain on paper towels and enjoy.

Pizza with Tomato and Cheese

Makes two 12-inch thin-crust pizzas

I've seen newly diagnosed people cry because they thought they had to say good-bye to their beloved pizza. But this recipe will convince you there is no need to do that. This dough is beautifully elastic thanks to the gum, the high protein flours, and the millet flour which gives it a chewy texture just like pizza should have. Use the toppings I've included or use your own.

There's no need to let this dough rise before baking. However, if you like a thicker crust, let it rise for 10 minutes before adding toppings and bake an additional 3 to 4 minutes.

1 cup white rice flour
¾ cup sorghum flour
¾ cup cornstarch or tapioca starch
½ cup millet flour
1 tablespoon xanthan gum
1 teaspoon salt

5 teaspoons instant active dry yeast
1⅓ cups warm water (110°F)
2 tablespoons olive oil
1 tablespoon honey
1 teaspoon cider vinegar
Cornmeal, to dust pans

CHEESE AND TOMATO TOPPING

3 teaspoons good-quality olive oil
8 tablespoons good-quality gluten-free pizza sauce
   (such as Muir Glen)
½ to 1 cup shredded mozzarella cheese, as desired
4 tomatoes, thinly sliced
⅓ cup freshly grated Parmesan cheese

▸ Preheat the oven to 450°F. Lightly oil two 12-inch pizza pans and dust with cornmeal. Set aside.

▸ In the bowl of a heavy-duty mixer fitted with the paddle attachment, beat the rice flour, sorghum flour, cornstarch, millet flour, xanthan gum, and salt together. Add the yeast and beat. Combine the water, oil, honey, and vinegar and add to the dry ingredients. Beat at medium-high speed for 3 to 5 minutes, or until the dough thickens.

▸ Scoop half of the dough onto a lightly oiled sheet of parchment paper. Cover with a sheet of lightly oiled plastic wrap. Use your fingertips and palms to lightly press the dough into a 12-inch circle. Flip the dough onto the prepared pizza pan and press to the edges of the pan. Use your fingertips to create a rim of dough around the edge to make a crust. Repeat with the remaining portion of dough.

▸ Divide the ingredients between the two crusts: Drizzle 1½ teaspoons of the olive oil over the surface of each crust. Top each crust with a light coating of pizza sauce and mozzarella cheese. Scatter the tomato slices and Parmesan over the top.

▸ Slide both pizzas onto the lowest rack in the oven (see note below) and bake for 20 to 24 minutes, depending on the thickness. The bottom of the pizza will be brown. Remove from the oven. Let cool slightly and slice.

Note: If your oven is small, make one pizza at a time. Or save half of the dough to use later. It can stay in the refrigerator overnight or can be frozen (in a ball or rolled out) for 4 weeks.

Sandwich Bread

Makes one 2-pound loaf

Finding a gluten-free bread with fiber, good taste, and texture is the ultimate challenge. Finding one that also makes a great sandwich is another story. This nutrient-dense bread is all of those and more. Use this for sandwiches at lunch or toast slices for breakfast. While the sunflower seeds add texture, they can be omitted.

If this becomes your go-to bread as it is mine, measure out all the dry ingredients (except the yeast) ahead. Mix and store the mixture in the refrigerator. When you have a hankering for bread, you'll just need to add the liquids and yeast.

1⅓ cups brown or white rice flour
¾ cup cornstarch or tapioca starch
¼ cup potato starch (not potato flour)
½ cup amaranth flour
½ cup millet flour
2 tablespoons brown sugar
1 tablespoon xanthan gum
1 teaspoon salt
⅓ cup roasted unsalted sunflower seeds
1 tablespoon instant active dry yeast
1 cup + 2 tablespoons warm water (about 110°F)
3 tablespoon honey
2 tablespoons olive oil
1 teaspoon cider vinegar
2 large eggs

▶ Lightly oil a 9-x-5-inch loaf pan.

▶ Combine the rice flour, cornstarch, potato starch, amaranth flour, millet flour, brown sugar, xanthan gum, and salt in the bowl of a stand mixer fitted with the paddle blade (or a medium-size mixing bowl). Add the sunflower seeds and beat well. Add the yeast and beat.

▶ In a separate bowl, combine the water, honey, oil, and vinegar. Add the eggs and beat to combine. Pour into the dry ingredients. Beat on medium speed for 3 minutes, or until the dough begins to pull away from the sides of the bowl.

▶ Scrape into the prepared pan. Smooth the top. Cover with oiled plastic wrap and let rise to the top of the pan (about 45 minutes). Preheat the oven to 350°F.

▶ Remove the plastic wrap and bake for 45 to 50 minutes, or until an instant-read thermometer reaches 200°F. Remove from the oven and turn out onto a rack. Let cool completely before slicing.

For Bread Machine

▶ Do not add the yeast to the dry ingredients. Place the liquid ingredients in the bottom of the bread machine baking pan. Sprinkle the dry ingredients over the liquids. Sprinkle the yeast over the dry ingredients. Close the top and set the bread machine on a gluten-free or shortest cycle (preferably with only one knead and one rise cycle) and press Start. Midway through the kneading cycle, use a rubber spatula to scrape down the sides and make sure all the flour is incorporated in the dough. When rise cycle begins, smooth the top of the dough. Once bread has baked, remove from the pan and allow to cool on a wire rack.

Soft Pretzels

Makes 12 pretzel twists

Dunking these in a baking soda bath, then baking them quickly at a high temperature lends the classic slightly crunchy veneer and chewy inside of a "real" soft pretzel. They are best eaten warm right from the oven, but are mighty tasty reheated the next day as well. Turn the dough into wonderful pretzel buns, too. Just form into rolls instead of twisting the dough into pretzels, let rise, follow the instructions for the baking soda bath, and then bake for 18 to 20 minutes.

1½ cups white rice flour
1 cup brown rice flour
¾ cup potato starch (not potato flour)
½ cup cornstarch or tapioca starch
2½ tablespoons packed brown sugar
3½ teaspoons xanthan gum
½ teaspoon salt
2¼ teaspoons active dry yeast

1½ cups warm milk
4 tablespoons unsalted butter
2 large eggs plus 1 yolk

BAKING SODA BATH

½ cup baking soda
8 cups water
Pretzel salt or coarse salt, for sprinkling

▶ Line two baking sheets with parchment paper and coat with vegetable spray. Set aside.

▶ In the bowl of a stand mixer fitted with the paddle attachment (or a medium-size mixing bowl), beat the white and brown rice flour, potato starch, cornstarch, brown sugar, xanthan gum, and salt together. Add the yeast and beat.

▶ Heat the milk with the butter until it reaches 110°F. Add to the dry ingredients, along with the eggs and egg yolk, and beat at medium speed for 3 minutes, or until the dough becomes smooth and pulls away from the sides of the bowl.

▶ Set a sheet of parchment paper on the counter and coat lightly with vegetable spray. Transfer the dough to the parchment paper and knead until smooth and coated with oil. Divide the dough into twelve pieces. Roll each into an 18-inch-long rope. Make a U-shape with the rope. Holding the ends, cross them over each other and press them onto the top of the rope to form a pretzel with three circles.

▶ Transfer to the prepared pans. Cover with lightly oiled plastic wrap while finishing the remaining pretzels. Preheat the oven to 425°F while the dough rises until nearly doubled in size, about 20 minutes.

▶ Meanwhile, make the baking soda bath. Heat the water in a deep skillet. When it begins to boil, add the baking soda. In batches, place the dough in the water and cook for 30 seconds on each side. Using a slotted spoon, transfer to the prepared pans and sprinkle with the pretzel salt right away so it sticks to the pretzels.

▶ Bake for 12 to 15 minutes, or until golden brown. Remove from the baking sheets and allow to cool on a rack for at least 5 minutes. Remove from the rack and eat warm or cool, and transfer to a resealable plastic bag and freeze. Reheat in a 400°F oven for 8 to 10 minutes. No need to thaw first.

PART THREE

Lifestyle
How to Go from Surviving to Thriving

Just a decade ago the landscape for a gluten-free life was far different than it is today. For one thing, very few people ate this way and most did so out of medical necessity. Physicians were reluctant to put people on the diet, viewing it as a life sentence instead of a lifestyle. It was too hard to follow, too limiting, and the food was terrible, they said. Indeed, there was some truth to that. As patients, we doubted we would ever eat "normally" again. Living well meant being hypervigilant in every aspect of our lives from restaurant dining to grocery shopping to traveling. Most products were not so delicious. I did a lot more baking and traveled with an extra suitcase filled with breads, crackers, and cereal, just in case.

Today physicians are more apt to recognize and test for diseases on the gluten intolerance spectrum—and they recommend the GFD regularly for reasons beyond celiac disease. And keeping pace with these medical advances, now there are great gluten-free products, with far more meal options than before. That said, while life is immeasurably easier and tastier, living well gluten-free is a regimen that permeates all aspects of daily life from dating and friendship to legal issues, health insurance and preexisting conditions, children's play groups, restaurant dining, home parties, travel, and more.

This section is the blueprint for a life well lived without gluten. It includes tips on explaining the diet to a server or a casual date, finding a good insurance carrier and a public restroom, and preparing for a hospital stay. In it, you will find coping skills and crucial everyday information.

What if you mistakenly eat gluten? Although there is no morning-after pill, no antidote, this section provides suggestions to make you more comfortable when you accidentally ingest gluten.

We'll talk about socializing, too. I'm big on it. I would never want you to miss out on a party or social gathering because you're afraid you won't find anything safe to eat. Dining out and traveling are outside the comfort zone for so many who need a gluten-free diet. Remember, the opposite of socializing is isolation. Socializing is especially critical when you are feeling lost in the gluten-free maze. Don't stay home and wallow in your gluten-free beer. We'll talk about how to get out, enjoy life, and take your special diet along. (And, yes, there is gluten-free beer—and you can have it along with your gluten-free pizza.) You'll find tips for explaining your diet to a host, and ideas for foods you can bring. From preventing cross-contamination on the grill to keeping croutons out of the salad to contributing a nutritious gluten-free dish that everyone can enjoy, it's all outlined here. Being fortified with this ammunition can make the difference between an enjoyable evening and one that creates anxiety.

If you are a parent of a child who is gluten-free, this comes with a whole additional set of concerns from Play-Doh to playdates. Having raised a son with celiac disease, I understand. And what about shared custody of a child who needs a GFD? How do you take joint responsibility for a diet? You'll find ideas and tips to help you, your child, and your family navigate this diet together.

If you are simply a gluten avoider, your level of vigilance on the diet depends on your reason for choosing to avoid gluten. We can still meet in the gluten-free bread aisle, but the subtle nuances of cross-contamination and an occasional apple pie are up to you. You'll find useful information in the sections on travel, attending parties, eating in restaurants, and even disaster preparedness and camping.

Whatever your reason for adopting a GFD, you'll discover tips to go from surviving to thriving. Come along. I'll take you there.

11

Getting Out
What You Need to Know to Eat and Travel Safely

Restaurants

A medical expert speaking at a celiac conference once said, "Eating in restaurants with celiac disease is like having unprotected sex." It's haunted me ever since. I have a love-hate relationship with restaurants. I love eating out, tasting new dishes, garnering new ideas for my own recipe writing. But I know that eating out can be risky business. Although I take every precaution imaginable, once in a while I wake up in the middle of the night with aliens playing hockey in my body, gnashing and slugging and poking at my insides. Some head for the mouth; others take a southerly route. And I know I've been gluten-ed. It's no secret. Eating in restaurants when you are gluten-free is like playing Russian roulette. You never know when you're going to encounter a difficult or inattentive server, a misinformed chef, or a line cook who's on his or her last day and truthfully, should have been gone yesterday.

But try not to get into a neurotic frenzy about this. Eating out is important to one's social life and I remain a huge advocate of restaurant dining. Social isolation might be nearly as harmful as gluten to a person's lifestyle. Armed with the best information, it's possible to minimize the dangers of restaurant dining and still have fun.

Wouldn't it be nice if every restaurant server was as knowledgeable about the menu's gluten-free options as about its nightly specials?

What's Behind Those Swinging Doors

While you sit comfortably at your table sipping a glass of wine, gluten-free beer, or a soda, and chatting with friends, a lot of activity is happening in the "back of the house," the place in restaurants that most of us never get to see. Understanding the back of the house helps minimize the risk of eating out.

First, select a restaurant where a chef is on duty and dishes are made to order. The chef is most likely to know all the ingredients in each dish. Ideally, have a face-to-face conversation, but if it's a busy time, an attentive manager can be the chef's best ambassador, the one who can act as the go-between and convey your concerns to the kitchen.

Second, ask the chef, manager, or server how gluten-free and other special-diet requests are tracked and recorded. Many restaurants have a "gluten-free" option in their system that's used when they place your order, or have another way of noting it in the computer. Some restaurants use different plates to let the cooks, server, and diner know that this meal has been prepared for a special diet. Other restaurants (and I love this one) have a sticky ticket that attaches to the lip of the plate and calls out the allergen.

Finally, know the areas where cross-contamination risks are the greatest so you can eat defensively. (For more questions to ask in a restaurant, see page 206.)

Six Dangerous Places in a Restaurant Kitchen

#1. Pasta Water: The Center Chimney in Many Restaurants

Before the evening service begins, a line cook sets a giant pot of water on the stove to boil. Pasta is cooked in this water all evening. By the end of the night, a thick, white, creamy sludge of gluten is suspended in the pot, like low-hanging fog. This is the water in which your gluten-free pasta could be cooked. It's also where a line cook might blanch a few stalks of broccoli or some green beans if the kitchen is running low on cooked veggies. And this water is used for other purposes as well. If a sauce or soup is too thick or the marinara is clumping, a cook might scoop out a ladle of this water to thin it. Since there's gluten in the water, it adds magnificent qualities to these, but not to you, if you eat it.

Remedy: Verify that gluten-free pasta is cooked in a separate pot and drained in a clean colander, or don't order pasta. Request that your sauce for a pasta dish be made separately in an area where spoons have not come in contact with regular pasta and pots of sauce.

Double-check that fresh vegetables will not be poached in the pasta pot.

#2. Fryer: Anything Goes Here, but You Should Not

Cross-contamination runs rampant in the restaurant fryer. Your order of French fries, even if they are safe, can pick up tidbits of fried clam batter, calamari, onion rings, or chicken nuggets, all favorites on restaurant menus.

Remedy: Unless a restaurant tells you it has a dedicated fryer for French fries or for gluten-free foods, **always avoid fried foods in restaurants**. You probably should anyway.

#3. The Salamander: Not the Amphibian Kind

Another centerpiece of a restaurant kitchen is the salamander, a metal box with a rotating shelf that passes by hot broiler coils. It is used for toasting and browning. Rolls and bread are set on the shelves. They pass the broiler coils at the back of the machine, then drop into a tray at the bottom of the machine, where a line chef removes them to fill orders.

The dumping tray gathers a trail of gluten crumbs throughout the day. If you simply ask your server to toast it, your gluten-free bread will land in that pile. Worse yet, your bread could sit there while gluten-filled rolls land on top of it. It is as creepy as having a mouse scamper across the table!

Remedy: Request that gluten-free bread be heated in the oven on a sheet of foil or microwaved on a paper towel. In fact, if any of the preparation for your order may involve browning or toasting, remind the server not to use the salamander.

#4. The Griddle: Diced, Scrambled, Tossed, and Grilled

Hamburger rolls, grilled cheese sandwiches, pancakes, and the like take form on the big slab of iron known as the griddle. This is rated #4 as it is not as chancy as the first three offenders. But depending on what is going on when your order is prepared, this one can be risky.

Remedy: Request that the area where your food will be grilled be scraped clean and that rolls and sandwiches are not grilled in the same area while your food is being prepared.

#5. The Pizza and Other Prep Areas

Restaurant kitchens are divided into sections. Cold and hot stations are in different parts of the kitchen. Salads and sandwiches are prepared in the first; sauté, frying, grilling, and pizza stations are in the hot area. Desserts are in another section of the kitchen and are mostly prepared ahead of time, meaning the pastry chef is probably not on duty when you have questions about dessert.

We've talked about grilling and frying. The sauté station is where your custom order will most likely be prepared. It's the safest area. Each dish should be prepared in a clean sauté pan with fresh ingredients. This is where you and the chef have the most control over your meal.

Not so with the pizza station. Even if pizza crust is rolled ahead, there's flour on each pan and in the air. In addition, ladles of sauce go between pizza dough and sauce container with regularity. Make sure your food is not prepped in this area.

Remedy: If the restaurant offers gluten-free pizza, make sure it's prepared in a location other than the pizza prep area (such as the salad station) and with clean utensils and fresh toppings. If it's baked in the pizza oven, make sure it's made in a separate, clean pan and baked on the top rack, or request that your pizza be baked in one of the regular (nonpizza) ovens.

#6. Soups and Sauces

Imagine yourself sitting in the front of the house, the dining area; the doors to the kitchen, a barricade between you and the place where your food is being prepared. In the stainless-steel turfdom, fine chefs and sous chefs are creating their sauces and soups, the flavorful additions that lend the signature to their work. Not unlike watercolors where a splash of green-blue, a touch of mauve to the sunset, add the distinct touches, sauces and soups are creations, too. And, like watercolors, they are complex composites made up of who-knows-what.

In addition to *who-knows-what* is a sprinkle of *chef prerogative*. If a sauce tastes a little bitter or doesn't have the flavor profile one night, he or she might add a little soy sauce or gravy booster. Is the chef going to admit that? Heck, no. Would you give away those little secrets?

Note: Soy sauce is added to the food in some Mexican restaurants and sometimes used in house-made Caesar salad dressings.

The same is true of soups. In addition, if the soup is too thin and evening service is beginning, someone might thicken the soup with flour, just a smidge. That's the last thing a gluten-sensitive person wants to hear.

Besides, many sauces and soups are thickened with a roux, a mixture of flour and butter.

It's also important to note that if you tell people you can't have wheat flour, many think you can still have "white" flour.

Remedy: Avoid all sauces unless you can verify with a chef that they are gluten-free.

Butter sauces (citrus or fruit, butter, and a splash or wine) are usually safe, as are cold sauces, such as those that are herb- or mayonnaise-based. They are less complex, usually easier to dissect, and less likely to need such random enhancements as a smidge of pasta water. Verify the preparation with the chef or manager before digging in.

Some soups are thickened naturally with vegetables and perhaps a splash of cream for enrichment. But these soups generally begin with vegetarian or chicken stock, so you'll need to know whether the stock is made in-house, or review the label if it's a commercial product.

Be sure pasta or barley is not added to the soup. I've encountered that surprise occasionally after doing all the detective work to dissect the composition of the dish itself. (Think: minestrone—sometimes it's made with pasta and sometimes it's not.)

Watch Out: When you ask a server what's in a sauce and he or she can only say, "It's okay. The chef thickens it with cornstarch." This may be an indication that the server does not have the full scoop on what's in the sauce, or your GFD, for that matter. It's time to pick something else, something simple, from the menu.

Bottom line: If you don't want a bunch of aliens taking over your body in the middle of the night, avoid soups and sauces unless you can be sure they are safe.

Seriously Gluten-free

Some people feel they just want to be gluten-free and think a little won't hurt.

—CHEF PETER POLLAY, CHEF-OWNER,
POSANA CAFÉ, ASHEVILLE, NC

People sometimes say they have a mild case of celiac disease. Isn't that like saying you're a little pregnant? You are or you are not. Celiac medical experts always remind us that even if we don't have symptoms, damage can still take place. But lately servers ask me whether I am "seriously gluten-free."

My flippant self wants to say, "Do you think I would be doing this if I didn't have to?" And I want to inform him or her that all gluten-free requests are serious. But I swallow my rhetorical questions. I realize that, to eat safely, the only response is, "Yes, seriously gluten-free. I have celiac disease and can't have a speck of gluten."

Then, the same person says, "I mean, do I need to change my gloves?" And I relax. He gets how serious this is. Now when I encounter a server in a restaurant who asks me if I am "seriously gluten-free," I nod and say, "Thank you for checking. Yes, it's a medical condition."

"It's just possible that the person served earlier in the evening was not as concerned about the diet as you are and that stirs up confusion in the hospitality industry," says Alice Bast, of the NFCA. "When a diner orders a gluten-free meal, what he or she often doesn't see is the extra time and cost that goes into preparing that meal—especially if the restaurant follows specific gluten-free safety protocols. Then, if that same diner orders a big slice of regular apple pie, it sends the kitchen the message that this is not a serious condition. It's frustrating for a restaurant that has gone out of its way to make things safe only to discover that the person doesn't need the diet, just likes to eat that way," says Bast.

It's frustrating for the seriously gluten-free diner, too. You simply can't know the protocol in place (or the restaurant's perception of its gluten-free diners' needs) until you've had a conversation, and have that dialogue, you must.

Gut Reaction: Gluten Envy

Don't think I don't notice when the server reaches past me with sleek wooden tongs, depositing slices of freshly baked bread on all the other bread plates.

"No, thanks." I wave my hand over the small plate to my left. Some meaningful friend who is sharing my table says, "She can't. She's gluten-free." She peers at me from around the pepper mill. "Poor Beth," she says as she breaks off a piece of her doughy delight and pops it into her mouth.

While announcing the specials, the server gracefully deposits a pool of green olive oil, a drizzle of balsamic vinegar, a few grinds of black pepper onto a communal plate.

Sometimes he tries to remove my bread plate. "I'd like to keep it," I say, brushing away his hand. "For sharing," I explain.

Someone says, "Sorry," as pieces of bread lounge in the olive oil. I don't know if that's regret about my diet, the fact that they are enjoying chewy, crusty loaves and I can't, or a way of apologizing for eating in front of me.

"I'm used to it," I say. But I'm totally *not*. If I had recorded all the times I had to go without—bread, pizza, pasta, doughnuts, pastry, birthday cake—I could write a book that is much longer than this one.

You probably know by now, I do not dwell on the negative parts of this diet. I'm usually more upbeat. But occasionally, a longing churns

▶

in my stomach, and I feel as abandoned as my bread plate. These are the times when I suffer from gluten envy.

I've watched without partaking for most of my life. As I child, I licked pats of butter off their paper as the rest of my family devoured rum biscuits or popovers. I entertained myself by building pyramids with single-serving cream containers while the others finished their pie à la mode.

These days, I live vicariously by asking my husband for his unbiased reviews. I know he can separate bread remorse from honest culinary appraisal. He describes the taste, the texture, dismissing a product as parbaked or stale, extolling the chew of the house-made Italian bread at one of our favorite restaurants. For that, I have lovingly dubbed him my seeing-eye pig.

Still, I fantasize about eating normally in a restaurant, sharing all the food that everyone else enjoys. I imagine a died-and-gone-to-heaven moment when I will be brought an entire gluten-free bread basket; just for me, a time when my husband, son, and I can have the same meals and enjoy, no, relish them.

And I've brushed up against this dream. At the American Celiac Disease Alliance annual meeting in Denver in 2007, we feasted at Panzano-Denver, where chef Elise Wiggins (herself wheat-free) cooked for us. Seating us around a huge table in the center of the dining room, a server placed a leather-bound menu in front of each of us. I opened the folder, preparing to analyze the dishes as I usually do. To my delight, the entire menu was gluten-free. I felt like a kid going out to eat for the first time. "All for us?" I asked.

I was still beaming when platters of Elise's famous gluten-free focaccia were set before us. I inhaled the first piece. For that night, my plate runneth over with gluten-free choices.

Today, gluten-free is moving closer to the center of the plate, and with it comes bread, gluten-free bread. At first, it wasn't so much an appreciation for the bread as being acknowledged, feeling somewhat normal, and having something to eat while everyone else feasted. But as my bread plate fills with choices, a feeling of inclusion sweeps over me, and I notice my gluten envy slipping away.

Grill the Server: Six Questions to Ask

- What's the protocol for handling a special diet?
- Does a manager or one single person follow my order from table to kitchen and back?
- Is my meal prepared in a clean pan with clean utensils?
- Is it served on dishes that differentiate my meal from the regular meals (e.g., round versus square plates)? Take note if others order the same dish, and your meal looks like theirs.
- Was it noted in the computer?
- Is a label attached to the plate to note that my meal is gluten-free?

If possible, call ahead before the restaurant becomes busy with lunch or evening preparations (ideally between two and five) and ask these questions of the manager or the chef.

Finally, where you sit matters: All these questions are useless if the server can't hear you. If you are farthest from the server and need to shout across the table in a noisy restaurant, it's difficult to make your special diet requirements heard. And it's even more difficult to hear the server's answer to your questions. Stake out a seat that puts you nearest your waiter or waitress. All bets are off if you are at a round table and the server takes the orders while standing in one place. You might need to leave the table to have that conversation.

Cross-Contamination: Every Crumb Matters

Remind your server to please have the kitchen:

- Scrape the grill before preparing your fish, hamburger . . . (you fill in the blank).
- Prepare your gluten-free pizza in a safe area free of gluten, and use separate sauces and utensils.
- Slice gluten-free bread or rolls with a clean knife and serve in a separate bread basket or on a separate plate.

- Prepare any other elements of your order fresh, using clean utensils, bowls, and pans.

It's a good idea to call ahead and address these issues when the kitchen is not busy. That way you'll have the chef or manager's undivided attention. The staff won't feel rushed and you won't feel that they see you as a whiny customer.

Diet Specifics: CD, GS, and GFBC

Celiac patients: All of the dining-out issues are critical for your diet. Cross-contamination can be as problematic as gluten itself, so question the restaurant staff thoroughly when placing your order.

Gluten sensitivity: Even crumbs of cross-contamination can make you sick. (That's why you avoid gluten.) Depending on the degree of reaction, grill your server as if you had celiac disease.

Gluten-free by choice: Steer clear of menu items that are wheat- and gluten-based. Avoid bread and select gluten-free pasta, if available. Otherwise, cross-contamination and small amounts of gluten may or may not mess up your evening. You decide.

Ways You Can Tell Whether a
Restaurant Takes Your Diet Seriously

- Does the restaurant have a gluten-free menu? That shows it's done some homework. Perhaps it has been vetted by one of the gluten-free training programs (page 206).
- Does the restaurant state "wheat-free tamari" on the menu? *If it lists "soy sauce" instead of wheat-free soy sauce or tamari, that might be a red flag.*
- Does the menu specify salad "without croutons" or "with gluten-free croutons"?
- Does the restaurant know the French fries are safe in and of themselves, *but* the fryer is shared and might cross-contaminate them?

- Does it offer gluten-free bread from a separate bakery or company and is it served separately from conventional bread? (If so, dig in. But don't let your fellow diners near your butter or dipping oil.)

It's not just those in the GF community who recognize the importance of restaurant awareness; foodies are taking note, too. Lisa Ekus is a literary agent and founder of the Lisa Ekus Group, where she works with many celebrity chefs. She's also the parent of a daughter with severe food sensitivities, including to gluten. Here's what she has to say about restaurants' responsibilities to their clientele:

"These days there's no excuse for restaurants not being fully educated about gluten-free options. The challenge is that so many people have chosen the gluten-free diet as a lifestyle, not a medical choice.

"Every request must be treated as a health issue. It's not for us to make the determination about the seriousness of someone's allergic reaction.

"I've watched for years as my daughter has doubled over in excruciating pain because she's been served something she can't have. This is not an option to be taken lightly."

Signs Your Dinner May Be in Danger

- The chef or server seems irritated by your questions.
- The server dismisses your questions and tells you not to worry. He or she knows all about your diet.
- The salad arrives with croutons that have not been specified "gluten-free." (Send it back and ask them to make it over. Remind them it's not okay to just pick out the croutons. *Be vigilant with every other item you order.*)
- The gluten-free bread comes in the bread basket with regular bread.
- The sorbet that's *safe* has a *real* cookie stuck in it and it's waving at you like a red flag.
- Several people handle the dish and it's served by a person you've never seen before.
- No one knows whether your order is gluten-free and the server does not indicate it when he or she brings your meal.

- You order the antipasto from the gluten-free menu and the server who is juggling six things, has a bread basket piled on top of it.

Ultimately it's up to you to know your own level of comfort or concern when you eat in a restaurant. It's okay to say, "No, thanks," and get up and leave if you feel uncertain your diet is in good hands.

In Defense of Food Service

You may have noticed an increase in the number of restaurants offering gluten-free options. It's not just you. According to an NPD Group market research company survey conducted in January 2013, nearly 30 percent of people are avoiding or cutting down on gluten in their diet. (Other market surveys say it's more like 20 percent, but that's still significant.)[1]

Chefs and restaurant personnel are also receiving training on handling food allergens in the restaurant kitchen. These programs include:

- Chef to Plate Gluten-free Restaurant Awareness Program run by Gluten Intolerance Group, gluten.net
- Gluten-free Food Service Management and Training Program (GFFS), a certification program run by Gluten Intolerance Group, gluten.net
- Gluten-free Resource Education Awareness Training (GREAT) program developed by the National Foundation for Celiac Awareness (NFCA), celiaccentral.org
- ServSafe, servsafe.com, a program of the National Restaurant Association and Food Allergy Research and Education (FARE), food allergy.org

And at least one state, Massachusetts, has mandatory food allergen training requirements.

Whether a restaurant is allergy aware or specifically gluten-free-friendly (GFF), this awareness helps ensure that the kitchen knows the ingredients and understands which are gluten-free. But don't get too relaxed. You can't count on every kitchen to know everything about your diet. You still need to be proactive to avoid being gluten-ed by proxy.

Restaurant Dining with Training Wheels

Take it slow. This is a one-person race. You are the winner, no matter how quickly you jump into the dining out scene after diagnosis. Familiarize yourself with the diet and give the gut time to heal before you go whole hog.

Start out with restaurants that you have been able to verify as GFF, either on their website or through a local support group. (Many national chains have a gluten-free menu and some also have kitchen protocol in place. This includes several fast-food chains, Wendy's, Chipotle Mexican Grill, and In-N-Out Burger among them. (See a complete list in the Resources, page 308.)

Do a dry run. Call the restaurant when it is not busy (between two and five p.m. is a good time to reach managers and chefs), and ask the questions on page 203.

When you go, enjoy the company. Sip a glass of wine or a gluten-free beer and imagine you are feeling normal again. Order something simple that you've selected ahead of time, thanks to your research.

After a few positive experiences, you'll be ready to loosen or remove those training wheels.

A Gourmand in Training

"Acquiring travel and dining savvy is a work in progress. Start with safe places like Disney properties for travel and local restaurants or chains that are known to be GFF for dining out. Develop a relationship with a local restaurant that you always loved and teach them how to be gluten-free. Test your own internal resources and see how comfortable you are in taking care of yourself. Practice saying, 'This is what I can eat,' until your comfort level makes it more pleasant than stressful to travel and eat out."

—LAUREN KOMACK, CREATOR OF "THE GLUTEN-FREE-WAY," A TRAVEL AND SUPPORT COLUMN SHE WRITES FOR THE *HEALTHY VILLI* NEWSLETTER

Restaurant Dining on Steroids

Once you are comfortable with the diet and the questions you need to ask, venture out to new restaurants. Check their website and review their menus to see which might be the most GFF. (A fish fry restaurant is not a good choice. It's a gluten frenzy of battered and fried food.) Call and speak to the chef or a manager during off hours. If you make a restaurant reservation using a system such as OpenTable, let the restaurant know you found it this way. It's a subtle way to convey that you will be reviewing them, too.

Most restaurants have some degree of understanding of the gluten-free diet. But you still need to determine whether their degree of understanding can accommodate a seriously gluten-free person or they just offer ingredients that are safe for gluten avoiders. (See page 203 for questions to ask.)

Pick a restaurant that has a chef in the kitchen and prepares everything from scratch. He or she will know all the ingredients in the food.

Avoid ethnic restaurants where language might be an obstacle in asking the right questions, or bring restaurant cards (see page 222 for more on restaurant cards) in that language to help bridge the communication gap.

Tips from a Seasoned Diner and Adventurer

Erin Smith is an adventurous gluten-free diner, traveler and founder of GlutenFreeGlobetrotter.com, GlutenFreeFun.blogspot.com, and Gluten-free MeetUp New York. Here's what she advises:

- Don't be shy about your condition. Conversation is the key to eating safely. Talk to the maître d', restaurant manager, and your server about your dietary needs. Look at these conversations as educating the staff about what eating gluten-free means to you and future patrons. Don't be rude, just be clear.
- Pick a restaurant that features a cuisine that is more gluten-free friendly. American steakhouses and Brazilian churrascarias are great options for

meat lovers. (Just check on sauces or gravies that accompany your meat.) Mexican, Southwestern, and Latin restaurants tend to serve corn-based dishes that are safe for the gluten-free diner. Organic and vegetarian restaurants usually have a good understanding of special dietary requests including gluten-free.

I use Erin's great tips myself and have found that Thai and Indian cuisines can also be GFF. Stay clear of soy and oyster sauce in the first and avoid breads and foods cooked in the tandoori oven (where breads are usually also baked) in Indian restaurants.

How to Pick a GFF Restaurant

Seasoned traveler Lauren Komack (see "Lauren's Story," page 223) offers these tips on locating safe restaurants when traveling or close to home:

- Determine the restaurant's real understanding of the diet by asking questions about food preparation and handling. Does it just offer gluten-free items or does the staff understand how to prepare the food safely, too?
- Select restaurants that are chef-owned. They are the friendliest and safest and more knowledgeable about all the ingredients used in their dishes.
- Chains with gluten-free menus are a good choice as they have an established protocol for handling special diets, but people can still get gluten-ed by server or kitchen mistakes.
- Places that have active celiac support groups tend to have cultivated personal relationships with restaurants and have educated the owners and chefs about the diet.
- Check out the reviews about a restaurant. You can gauge the GFF level by reading comments. They'll tell you whether the restaurant really caters to special diets or has minimal options.
- Check out the restaurant's website. If it has a gluten-free menu or clear notations on the regular menu, it probably has more awareness.

Restaurant Resources:
Places to Check for GF-Friendly Restaurants

For information on locating GF-friendly restaurants and a list of popular restaurants that are GF-friendly see Resources, page 308.

FDA Gluten-free
Labeling Rule and Restaurants

Sink your teeth into this. The new FDA rule directs restaurants making the gluten-free claim to follow the same guidelines established for packaged foods, including the less than 20 ppm of gluten threshold. It's unclear how this will work or the impact it might have on restaurants offering gluten-free menu items. As this book went to press, restaurants were already switching to terms like, "menu for our gluten-sensitive diners" or "gluten-free friendly." You'll still need to grill the server to dine safely.

A Catered Affair

I love it when an invitation arrives and it says, "Please let us know if you have any special diet needs." But that rarely happens. What's more, many of us assume a party menu is fixed and cannot be modified. We just hope we'll find something to eat at the event.

According to Tracy Stuckrath, president of Thrive! Meetings and Events, a majority of the time planners don't ask whether anyone needs a special meal, which diminishes the opportunity to provide the guest with something to eat that is tasty and will not harm him or her. Besides, if the request is last minute, at the event itself, it really throws off the kitchen.

Not only is it okay, but a good idea to make your request for a special meal known. If you have to sit there and watch everyone else eat, it can be a long evening. Besides, the planner/caterer and the host want you to have a good time. Here are some tips to help you enjoy a safe, gluten-free affair.

Who to Contact

The first point of contact should be the host. Mention your dietary needs and ask whether there is a process to accommodate such needs. If not, ask whether it's okay to contact the caterer. Get the name and phone number. Give the caterer a call and ask what is being served. Some caterers have a website with menu options and describe how they handle special diets. That gives you a starting point when you speak, but know that most caterers customize event menus for each client.

What if you can't reach the host? Call the facility where the event will take place and ask who is catering the Jones affair on May 16. Depending on the venue, the caterer may be in-house or you might have to call another company. The caterer will let you know in the unlikely event that it needs the host's approval to accommodate your diet.

The caterer orders the food well ahead. *Call at least 72 hours and preferably one to two weeks prior to the affair.* This allows time to build your needs into the overall plan. Discuss simple changes: steak with no sauce or chicken without gravy; a baked potato in place of pasta; and a portion of salad without croutons.

The caterer might not be able to provide gluten-free bread and crackers. So, bring your own.

Set Up a Point Person and Card System

Tracy suggests some great ways to create a personal point of contact that can heighten your level of comfort when you arrive at the event. She recommends asking the planner to designate a server who will help handle your meal and will not touch any of the other meals until yours has been served. Ask to be introduced to that person upon arriving at the event and see whether he or she could wear a different color apron or bow tie or hat, so you can spot him or her if you have questions during the event.

Ask whether the meeting planner can use cards to delineate your meal from others. If he or she is amenable, ask the person to create two cards saying "gluten-free" or the specific food you need to avoid—one to put on the table where you will be seated and another for the kitchen to put on top of your meal.

Kids and Events

Tracy's tips are especially helpful if kids are attending a party without adults. Usually this happens when the kids are young teenagers attending friends' bar or bat mitzvahs or Sweet Sixteen–type parties. With the help of the party planner, designate one staff person at the event who will serve as the liaison for your child. Perhaps he or she can wear a purple baseball cap or a red bandana that lets your child know this is the person in charge of his or her meal. Coordinate the details ahead of time so you can relax knowing your kid will have a worry-free, gluten-free time. If your child allows you to walk with him or her into the venue, seek out the party planner and staff person and introduce yourself and your child.

If your child is a teenager, good luck getting past the door with him or her in tow. You'll pull up to the curb, drop your child, and come back after the party ends. You will have to trust that your teen will seek out the right people. But you have a chance to rehearse the scenario at home and once again in the car on the way to the event.

Hit the Road: Travel in the United States

Gluten-free-Friendly Cities

> Once one restaurant offers a serious gluten-free menu, and other restaurants see how successful they are, others follow suit. Once people find us, they eat here every meal. You can get a customer for life and in a tourist town, word gets out. It's great for business.
>
> —Peter Pollay, chef-owner, Posana Café, Asheville, NC

Asheville, North Carolina, is a mecca for gluten-free diners. Leading the way is Posana Café, run by chef-owner Peter Pollay whose wife was diagnosed with celiac disease a few years ago. But many midsize cities have successfully captured the gluten-free market. While larger cities tend to have good gluten-free resources and choices, don't overlook these smaller urban areas.

Here is a partial list of cities that are known for having many GFF restaurants. By the time you read this book, the list will have doubled, no doubt.

- Asheville, North Carolina
- Austin, Texas
- Boston, Massachusetts
- Boulder, Colorado
- Charleston, South Carolina
- Chicago, Illinois
- Denver, Colorado
- Eugene, Oregon
- Napa, California

- New York, New York
- Orlando, Florida
- Portland, Oregon
- Sanibel Island, Florida
- San Francisco, California
- San Jose, California
- Seattle, Washington
- Sonoma, California
- Washington, DC

Disney—Not Just for Kids

Disney properties and cruise lines are known for accommodating gluten-free travelers, with an abundance of options and often have a concierge service set up to handle special diet requests.

Planning a Trip

Skipping a meal because you can't find safe food, or ending up sick because you took a risk can ruin your travel plans. Some advance research on your destination can help avoid these circumstances and make your trip run smoothly.

- Look for natural food markets, Trader Joe's, large supermarkets, and Whole Foods Market locations in the area.
- Book a hotel with a kitchen or at least a refrigerator.
- Pick a hotel with knowledge of the GFD. (Marriott, Ritz-Carlton, Omni, and Fairmont are some chains that accommodate GFD.)

- Look up the local support group's website. It's likely to offer restaurant and shopping tips (see page 308 for some great online resources).
- Pack your own bread, crackers, breakfast cereal, and snacks. Pick durable foods so they don't turn to crumbs en route.

Taking the Scenic Route (Rural America)

Traveling to small towns, rural locations, and national parks tends to provide an abundance of vistas and views. But gluten-free travelers and diners may have difficulty locating restaurants or even stores that offer safe choices along the way. This is where your resourcefulness shows. Pack bread, cereal, snacks, and nutrition bars so you can spend your time enjoying the scenery and not hunting for food. Find a natural food store that is on your route and call to make sure it carries gluten-free items. Do an Internet search for grocery stores in the location of the park or town where you will be staying. If you are heading to a national park, the Park Service or website for that park can let you know which nearby grocery stores have gluten-free options. Most national parks offer gluten-free selections in food service locations within the parks.

Getting the Most out of Gluten-free Travel Research on the Internet

Joel is board certified in emergency medicine. He is also my husband and a great gluten-free travel planner. Since no amount of medicine can help my son or me when we have a gluten reaction, his research in advance of our trips is invaluable. Most of his information is gathered from the Internet, where he has learned to slog through hundreds of sites to find the plums that are GFF and enjoyable for all of us.

His attitude: travel should be adventurous, fun, relaxing, and free of gluten reactions. He plans our travel this way:

- Enter "gluten-free travel" in a search engine.
- Pick websites that have filters allowing you to select locations and places to eat that are friendly to your diet.

- TripAdvisor and OpenTable list gluten-free restaurants by location. Travel blogs are helpful, too.
- Search for the location plus "gluten-free."
- Search for the name of the inn or restaurant plus "gluten-free."
- Search for local or regional magazine and newspaper websites, and then for articles on gluten-free.

Follow-ups:

- E-mail the restaurant or inn in advance, particularly if you are traveling internationally. If you don't speak the local language, get some help writing the message in the native language. Restaurant cards are invaluable for this. (For more on restaurant cards, see Resources, page 309.)
- Do your part to help others. Write reviews on travel websites. Include specific comments regarding gluten-free so these will be available to other gluten-free travelers and will get picked up by search engines. Compliment restaurants that are doing a good job serving gluten-free customers.

Tips:

- Read the newest comments first, as the hospitality industry is always changing.
- Always put your gluten-free request into your e-mail reservation for an inn or restaurant.
- If you e-mail a restaurant or inn about your requirements and it doesn't reply, move on.
- Take the e-mail response with you so you have the name of a real person (frequently the owner, chef, or manager) whose name you can drop, or who might be present to help you navigate the menu.
- Beware of certain food websites that have long lists of "gluten-free-friendly" restaurants without any details or travelers comments, as the information may be incomplete, inaccurate, or old.

- Learn all you can about the local diet so you can ask the right questions; for instance, if you know the basic ingredients of paella, you can narrow your questions to "Do you use only arborio rice?" and "Do you make your own chicken stock?"
- Stay clear of restaurant buffets. Unless a chef can walk you through the selections and point out the safe foods, buffets are gluten traps. And eat carefully from salad bars, selecting only fresh individual items and avoiding mixtures of ingredients, such as potato salad, or items that sit next to croutons and other gluteny foods.

Inns and Outs of Traveling Gluten-free

- We stay in small inns and B & B's whenever possible. Our favorites (researched by Joel) are those where we get to know the owners and they get to know my diet. But the kitchens are beehives of activity during breakfast, and although they take my needs very seriously, I still worry about cross-contamination. I fear a summer hire is in the back room, stirring my blueberry pancakes with the same spoon he or she has just used to mix everyone else's pancakes or that the gluten-free crackers for evening wine tasting are stored in the same container as the gluten-filled crackers. So I devised a checklist for the owners. I e-mail all or part of this list after determining how receptive they are to my diet. If the inn has talked about its commitment to a GFD on its website, mention this as a way to break the ice. Also be sure to mention something like, "I am so appreciative that you are willing to provide me with a gluten-free meal." This is a great lead-in to: "Here are a few things I need to tell you about my diet":
  - Gluten-free is not just about the ingredients. It's about handling and preparation, too. Even crumbs of wheat that mingle with gluten-free food can make me ill.
  - Imagine this is raw chicken. It should not touch foods that are not going to be cooked or cutting areas that are not sanitized first. *Similar mindful precautions are appreciated in handling my gluten-free food.*
  - Store gluten and gluten-free products separately as crumbs can comingle.

- Please don't serve my gluten-free food in the same bread basket as gluten-filled baked goods, or my crackers in the same bowl
  with gluten crackers.
- Please use separate spoons for preparing or scooping batter, and
  clean knives for cutting gluten-free bread. (Beaters, muffin tins,
  cookie sheets, can be contaminated, too. But gluten can be removed by washing them carefully in warm soapy water.)
- Sponges used to wipe flour from a counter can spread gluten.
  (Paper towels work well.) If all else fails, I am happy with plain
  eggs, an omelet (from fresh eggs), plain yogurt with fresh fruit,
  or commercially prepared gluten-free cereal, and store-bought
  gluten-free bread (toasted in a clean toaster, please).

Overall, be gracious, but concerned. You can always ask for plain eggs
and bring your own bread that can be warmed in the oven. But if they
balk, pick another, more GFF place. Mindset matters.

Camping

Take a look at "Disaster Plan, Take 2," on page 280, and you might see
some similarities between camping and that section. The supplies, even
some of the transportation tips, are the same. The difference? You call the
shots, not nature. If you need ice, you can find it. A hot shower, a warm
meal—all easy to come upon. Hiking and backpacking are even closer.
Take a look at the grab-and-go survival kit preparations discussed on page
285. This should be old hat to you.

Camping, backpacking, and hiking when you have food allergies or
need a GFD are some of the easiest things to do. Many camping foods are
gluten-free (take a look at page 315 in the Resources section). In addition,
you can preplan everything; you can design your meals around your needs
and taste. Besides, you've got your food with you so you are never going to
go hungry.

In addition, you can add fresh eggs, fresh meats, cream for coffee, milk,
cheese, and gluten-free bread to your menu, depending on the availability
of ice or refrigeration.

Bonus: Many of these foods can be taken through TSA security so they are perfect for long trips and international journeys, too.

International Travel—Gluten Tag!

GFF Countries (partial list)

Australia	Israel
Great Britain	Mexico
Greece (see note below)	South America (corn-based cuisine)
Ireland	Spain
Italy	Turkey

Note: Beware the flour wars. While Greece can be great for GF travelers, there's one day a year you'll want to stay clear. Every Ash Monday, revelers in the Greek port town of Galaxidi participate in a flour war marking the end of carnival season and the beginning of the forty-day Lent period until the Orthodox Greek Easter. They celebrate by tossing flour at one another, drinking (of course), and partying. But this would not be much of a party for someone on a gluten-free diet. Wait until the festivities are over before visiting Galaxidi.

Most Difficult Countries to Visit

Language and cuisine make these challenging countries to visit. Book a tour with a guide who is knowledgeable about both.

China
Ethiopia
Kenya
Korea
Pakistan
Russia
Rwanda

Airlines: the Unfriendly Gluten-free Skies

Gluten-free airline travel might be the ultimate oxymoron. While gluten-free has taken off in all other sectors of food service, it has crash-landed when it comes to the airline industry. You're lucky to get peanuts instead of pretzels on a domestic flight and half the time the peanuts are coated with wheat starch (read the label before eating). Couple this with the fact that TSA limits the food you can bring through security *and* most airports are notoriously bad about offering gluten-free options in their food concessions. It's downright unappetizing to fly these days. But, hey, we are not cavemen and fly we must if we want to explore the world or attend a business meeting.

International travel might be a little easier than domestic air travel as most airlines expect to feed travelers on these long flights and many offer a gluten-free meal option as part of that service. I'd like to say that you can select that option when you book your flight, even if it's online. And half the time, I'd be right and you would get that meal.

But it's lonely at 35,000 feet. Flight attendants are onboard for your safety, but suffice it to say they are not there for your gut safety. They have no clue what's in the food they serve. It's prepared by a contracted caterer. The meals arrive with simple labels, such as "gluten-free" or "meat" or "chicken," that might become separated from the meal. Your meal can get served to the wrong person or might not make it onto the flight. You're halfway to London when you discover something amiss with the food you ordered and there is no one to ask, nothing to eat.

Some airlines may be better equipped to handle a gluten-free meal in first class or business class than in coach. And some foreign carriers (e.g., British Airways and Lufthansa) may be better able to handle special diets. But this is all speculative and based on a few travelers' comments. Besides, airline policies change more frequently than their in-flight movies.

Fortify Yourself

When you book your flight, speak with an agent and ask him or her to read the description of the gluten-free entrée you are likely to receive. At least you will be able to steer clear if you are served beef and were told to expect chicken.

Part of the food service routine might be to add a roll or slices of bread to each tray. Do not assume that "added" bread is also gluten-free. Unless it is prepackaged and labeled, don't touch it.

Disaster Planning, Take 1

I hate to be a Debbie Downer, but when it comes to airline travel, you need to plan for a worst-case experience and bring your own snacks and food on the plane. If the food served is safe, you can keep your stash for another time.

TSA

You've probably noticed the "no-liquids-and-gels" policy that limits what food you can bring through Transportation Security Administration (TSA) security checkpoints.

Most solid foods are okay. Here are a few ideas:

- Fruit
- Veggies
- Salad (Pick up dressing or condiments in an eatery once you pass through TSA or dress your salad right before you leave home.)
- Sandwich (Spreads are okay here.)
- Cookies
- Brownies
- Pretzels
- Chips
- Crackers
- Cereal
- Granola and granola bars

The following foods are not allowed (unless they are 3 ounces or less); many (larger-size products) can be picked up in eateries after you pass through TSA.

- Nut butters (unless spread on a sandwich)
- Hummus (unless spread on a sandwich)
- Salsa
- Yogurt
- Drinks
- Salad dressing
- Preserves

TSA allows drinks and liquids that are "medically necessary," along with prescription and OTC medications in any quantity. But you may need a note or prescription from the doctor specifying that these are medically necessary.

Once you pass through TSA security, most airports have few, if any, gluten-free options. You are lucky to find a bag of plain potato chips, yogurt without granola topping, or fruit salad. But this aspect of air travel is improving. Lately, gluten-free menus are appearing at many airport eateries. At the very least, look for chain restaurants—Wolfgang Puck, Au Bon Pain, Legal Seafood, Wendy's, and McDonald's—all of which have some gluten-free options (see a list of fast-food chains on page 308). But don't discount the local eateries in airports. Often they are better at offering gluten-free food, thanks to the influence of local celiac support groups. You'll find good choices at Baltimore Washington Airport, Chicago's O'Hare, Dallas–Fort Worth, Denver, Miami, San Francisco, and Washington National/Reagan Airport, to name a few.

The difficulty is that even if you do the research, you have no way of knowing where your flight will land or take off. The eatery with a gluten-free menu could be clear across the airport.

Once You Land

In addition to snacks and bars for the plane trip, pack items in your luggage for backup during your visit.

- Crackers
- Gluten-free bread, preferably vacuum sealed to extend the shelf life

- Granola and granola bars
- Snack bars
- If you are lactose and dairy intolerant, bring a good supply of Lactaid pills, but check the labels, as some are not gluten-free.

Toaster Bags

Whoever invented these is brilliant. Toast-It Reusable Toaster Bags and Toastabags reusable bags allow you to toast bread in a communal toaster without fear of cross-contamination. These are perfect not only for hotels and breakfast buffets, but also for office lunch and dorm rooms, and let you enjoy toast and sandwiches when you travel. You can buy these on several websites.

How to Say That: Restaurant Cards in Many Languages

Restaurant cards exist in every conceivable language and are a helpful way of explaining your diet when traveling to other countries—or eating in ethnic restaurants in the United States where the food is wonderful, but the English is not. A card written in the language of the person who is preparing your meal takes the worry out of communicating your needs and lets the restaurant know you are serious about this diet. (Bring a few copies of the card when you travel. Your server might forget to give it back.) See Resources, page 309, for where to obtain restaurant cards.

Lauren's Story:
Separating the Wheat from the Chef

Lauren Komack was rediagnosed with celiac disease in 1989. A seasoned travel before diagnosis, she has not let her diet come between her and a passion to explore the world. Turkey, Egypt, Jordan, Thailand, Guatemala, Brazil, Honduras, Vietnam, Cambodia, Italy, Ireland, the United Kingdom, and France are just a few of the "stamps" in her passport.

Lauren's pick-up-and-go attitude began when she and her late husband traveled. "I would print out the restaurant card in the appropriate language and off we went. I never had any problems or worries. I sought out places to eat that had a chef in the kitchen or, even better, where the owner was the chef. They could tell me what's okay and what to avoid."

She writes a travel and support column for the *Healthy Villi* newsletter, a very active celiac support group serving the Boston area.* As a licensed psychotherapist, Lauren combines her interest in helping people live well with celiac disease with teaching timid travelers and wary diners ways to take charge of their diet.

"Some people are afraid to say anything if they are served a meal that doesn't look quite right," she says. "Others are afraid to talk to the chef or don't know what to ask," continues Lauren. "As long as you take a friendly approach and are clear about the message that you'll get sick if you eat gluten, I've found that people are very helpful."

Her philosophy is that each person needs to find their own comfort zone. "Build your internal skills and learn how to become your own advocate. Find that place where you can comfortably tell people you need to eat gluten-free." To do that, she says it's important to understand how the food is prepared in the countries you are visiting. For instance:

- In Turkey, the lentil soup is made with bread crumbs.
- In Greece, where most of the food is GFF, the chicken soup known as avgolemono might contain orzo (pasta) and the saganaki (traditional flaming cheese) contains flour or bread crumbs.

▶

▼

- Some places, such as Israel and Australia, have entire restaurants and stores that are gluten-free. But in Israel, the falafel is often made with wheat.
- In Italy, pharmacies are well stocked with gluten-free products.

When traveling to more exotic locations, book guided tours and let the guide negotiate all the meals, says Lauren, who has used Overseas Adventure Travel (oattravel.com) for many of her trips.

On tours, "I check in with the tour guide at each meal and ask what I can eat. The guide walks through the menu or buffet with me so I know what is safe."

For cruises, she recommends contacting the cruise line when booking a trip. "The minute I check in and put my luggage in the room, I head to the dining hall to confirm my dietary needs with the chef. And then I check in again when I go to dine."

Her ultimate trip: a safari where everything was made on an open fire, including her gluten-free bread.

---

*The *Healthy Villi* is now the New England Celiac Organization (NECO).

12

Socializing

The Emotional Toll of a Special Diet

Food and socializing go hand in hand. All those holidays shared with family, Thursday night get-togethers with pizza and beer, picnics, and barbecues. Well, now they are sprinkled with special diet needs and a disconnect that comes with leaving behind all those wonderful foods you always associated with these events. And those coping mechanisms change with every age.

As children, it's trying to be normal and in control even though we feel neither. As teenagers, it's more about denial and perhaps even depression or rebellion. The overarching emotion is: *Why do I have to be different?* Young adults are dating and preparing for college, stressful times without adding the GFD. As adults, we might have developed more resilience and know-how and are fortified with safe solutions that we bring to our daily routine. But then, if we are raising children and teenagers, that adds another level of complexity.

Like the issues of coping with a special diet, this chapter, too, is complex. We'll discuss school and sleepovers, bullying, preparing for college, even how to play Beer Pong without beer. And I'll offer coping skills and tips to help you go from surviving to thriving.

If you're gluten-free by choice, you might face another set of conflicts, that of convincing others you really mean it when you say "gluten-free." "Just a little won't hurt this one time" is a comment you'll often hear.

It's like being chicken-ed when you are vegetarian. When you choose to be gluten-free, you may find your plate is filled with more than just rice cakes.

Kids and the GFD

Imagine being the kid at the birthday party who can't eat the cake. The *one* left out of the end-of-year pizza party in school. The *only* kid who reads labels on Halloween candy before trading with friends or has to ask the waitress questions before he orders. Celiac kids are thrown into complex social situations all the time. Who else can read and understand such terms as *hydrolyzed protein* or *modified starch* at the age of six?

Perhaps your child spent years feeling ill. This new diet has brought him or her back to health, but at what cost to friendships and routines?

As a parent, it's your job to support and guide your child while teaching him or her how to make healthy choices that will last a lifetime. You juggle everyone's needs—those with gluten issues and those without. And you keep smiling, although a feeling of guilt washes over you from time to time and you ask, "Why can't my child be like everyone else?"

Candid Kids—What Parents Should Know

When kids share candid perceptions of their own special diet, these invaluable insights help us all better understand how our own kids cope with the GFD in their world. These comments were recorded on a wonderful video presented by Boston Children's Hospital, childrenshospital .org. It was created by Tracy Keegan, a mother who raised two celiac children. Take a look at some of what they say.

- I just want to have what the other kids have.
- I was afraid I wouldn't fit in.
- Gluten-free food is an acquired taste. I'm getting used to it now.
- I'm not on *that* kind of diet.
- Kids say my food is from Mars.
- As long as I have something to eat, I don't feel left out.

Gut Reaction: The Inheritance

Revised from a piece called "Mother's Guilt," that appeared in Living Without, *August/September 2010*

As a protective older mother, I sought the best for my only child. I made sure he had lots of attention, a good education, wholesome food, music lessons, swimming instructions, travel experiences—any indulgence we could afford. I passed down my traditions, explained his place on the family tree and shared jokes about our eccentric relatives. I made sure he wore a helmet when he rode his bicycle and I covered him with shin and elbow pads when he skateboarded. But as much as I tried to protect him, I couldn't prevent him from getting celiac disease. Like me, he needs to be on a gluten-free diet for life.

Usually I'm a glass-half-full person, especially when it comes to having celiac disease. I dwell on what I can have rather than what I can't. But when it came to my child, I sometimes found myself peering out from the bottom of the glass. When he was young, I devoted countless hours to making sure he was never singled out, that he didn't have to compare his special-diet fare with the foods his friends were eating.

I orchestrated every food opportunity I could possibly control. His Sunday school class made braided challah so I improvised a gluten-free recipe so he could braid and eat with them. And I volunteered to teach the class so I could supervise his preparation without appearing to hover.

When his class had birthday parties, I found out what the birthday child's mom was bringing in and made something identical (or close to it) in a gluten-free variation. I was so grateful to the parent who asked if she could make something gluten-free that I bought the mix for her to use and gave her several pages of instruction. It broadened my son's support team and mine when someone else acknowledged his diet and embraced it.

During his teens, I really sparkled at the kids' pizza parties. By then I had discovered that "normal" packaging could trick everyone into thinking there was no special diet. When my son was invited to a

▶

▼

party, not only did I make a gorgeous pizza with pepperoni slices positioned just like Pizza Hut's, I ran to the local pizza shop for a printed box.

The box was a good trick that I played often. I tucked homemade cupcakes, cookies, and brownies into the ubiquitous white baker's boxes in order to get everyone's seal of approval.

When my son went off to college, I could no longer oversee his diet or his life. I could not run into New York City to bring him a gluten-free sandwich or a pizza or a cake. I had to release my grip and trust that he had the tools he needed, that he had inherited my genes for survival as well as the ones for celiac disease.

To my surprise, he's ended up very well adjusted. He cooks for himself. He orders in restaurants. He is healthy.

In the stillness of his absence, an insight has surfaced along with a morsel of regret. *How much of my frenetic hovering was due to self-blame for giving him this disease?*

He's a grown man, comfortable with the gluten-free lifestyle and empowered by his disease—monitoring his diet, understanding his body, committed to his own wellness.

Nevertheless, watching him from afar, that spot of guilt sometimes resurfaces . . . just for a moment. And then I reflect on our gene pool, grateful to have also given him tenacity, a sense of humor and an appreciation for safe, gluten-free food.

- I can trust my friends. They won't make fun of me. But I don't tell many other people about my diet.
- When I tell people, they ask too many questions.
- Look how many people have gone through this and they are normal—famous athletes, doctors, actors, and stuff.
- I feel like every other kid. I just have to eat differently.

To empower our kids means doing the research and empowering ourselves first. Here are a few tips to get you started:

- Check the celiac websites (page 303).
- Sign up for the Celiac Listserve (page 303).
- Stockpile good gluten-free foods.
- Adapt your kitchen and embark on gluten-free cooking.
- Find a Raising Our Celiac Kids (ROCK) group near you, by searching the Internet for the keywords "raising our celiac kids" plus your location (for more on ROCK, see page 230).
- Contact a local support group. Many have a kids' group affiliated with them.
- Start your own informal age-appropriate group: a play group for smaller kids, bowling parties for older kids, etc.
- Get local contact information from your child's physician or a children's hospital in your area. (Links are available through the national support group websites [see Resources, page 301] and search engines.)
- Involve the whole family. Your child's condition is everyone's issue. (In fact, you really won't be able to avoid this.)
- Volunteer for causes related to this diet and lifestyle.

The Key Is to Get Your Child Involved

- As soon as he or she is old enough, grocery shop together.
- As soon as your child can read, teach him or her to read labels.
- Role-play situations where the child needs to ask a parent, a sitter, a teacher, or a cafeteria person whether something is safe to eat.
- Encourage your child to write an essay or a poem about the diet or celiac disease or gluten sensitivity.
- When the child is young, create a play with other members of the family and make gluten the villain.
- Have the child do a cooking demonstration in school or camp, or make a gluten-free bread and share it with peers.
- Incorporate gluten, gluten sensitivity, and celiac disease into science fair projects.

Kids ROCK

Adults on a GFD understand the importance of social support and draw on a reserve of coping mechanisms that comes from years of experience. But kids, depending on the age at diagnosis, don't have all those coping skills. The simple act of sharing a birthday cake or a pizza can set up social and emotional barriers. The more aware parents are of the potential obstacles, the better the emotional well-being of the child. ROCK (Raising Our Celiac Kids) and other support groups aimed at children can help create a safe environment in which to enjoy the company of peers and practice skills that work in other situations. As the chapter leader of the Long Island ROCK Group, Randi Albertelli knows these simple strategies all too well.

Randi founded the ROCK group after her daughter was diagnosed with celiac disease in 2005 at the age of five. When the rest of the family was tested, Randi and her husband were both diagnosed. Only their son does not have the disease. "He eats the bread basket when we go out," says Randi.

Because of the local group and family support, Randi says that celiac disease has been only a positive force in their lives. "Our children have a certain resiliency that makes them who they are because of this diet. It's part of my daughter's persona. At her age I am not sure I would have the confidence to ask to read the ingredients at someone's house," says Randi. But the ROCK kids have mastered this as well as the questions to ask when they eat in restaurants.

ROCK-LI, rockli.com, runs bowling parties and scavenger hunts as well as safe gluten-free pizza get-togethers. And it works with the schools in its area to increase awareness about the diet and how it affects their kids. The organization is also trying to change the way schools think about bringing food to every celebration. But it's an uphill battle. "People have trouble changing; kids expect a birthday cake is necessary for every birthday," Randi says. "Creating events that do not revolve around food can be challenging."

From Play-Doh to Play Group and Beyond

What do spontaneity and the gluten-free diet have in common? Not so much, I'm afraid.

Even if your child is new to this diet, you've probably already noticed you can't pick up a grab-and-go meal for the family the way you did before-gluten-free. Although planning gets easier the longer you live in the realm of the gluten-free, you'll always need a game plan.

If you take a road trip and all the kids want a snack, stopping in a rest area might be the perfect solution for two, but will it provide a safe treat for your kid with gluten issues?

Perhaps soccer practice ran late. Ordinarily you might pick up a pizza or take-out Chinese. You'll need to broaden those choices a bit to snare some gluten-free options in your net. (Think Thai or Indian, instead; you may want to have a few go-to local restaurants that know you and your family. When you call and say it's Sally Smith, they'll know it's "Sally Smith with the GF order.")

And trying to keep the peace means feeding everyone, equally, with good safe foods. You can't leave someone out, after all, or feed them something they don't like because they can't have the gluten-filled pizza. We talked about easy meal options in Part 2, but with kids, there are often parties and playdates; here are some suggestions to manage those.

Celebrate

Nothing says "celebration" like a party that involves everyone and lots of yummy choices. With a few options and a bit of flair, you can turn any event into a celebration that will earn you points with your family and your children's friends. Try these for starters.

BURGER BONANZA
- Fill squirt bottles with mustard, ketchup, barbecue sauce, or other favorite condiments.
- Let each person decorate his or her own burger (chicken, turkey, beef, or veggie).
- Have plenty of gluten-free buns on hand for everyone.

CEREAL PARTY
- Many cereals are gluten-free.
- Fold in melted marshmallows or peanut butter and chocolate that have been melted together.
- Put out a stack of bowls, some cut-up fruit, and revisit breakfast. (This makes a great pajama party.)

MINI CUPCAKE DELIGHTS
- Buy a gluten-free cake or cupcake mix and make mini cupcakes.
- Use colorful cupcake papers to line the pans and have the kids scoop the batter into the paper-lined pans. Bake them and let them cool.
- Make a batch of confectioners' sugar frosting.
- Scoop the frosting into many bowls and set out food coloring.
- Let each child add his or her favorite color to a bowl until you have a rainbow of colors to pick from.
- Spread out bowls of M&M's or crushed peanut butter cups or other gluten-free decorations.
- Let everyone decorate several cupcakes. (Freeze extras, unfrosted, for another party.)

HIDDEN TREASURE PARTY
- Make up a gluten-free cupcake or muffin mix. Line a muffin pan with cupcake papers.
- Half-fill each muffin cup with batter.
- Have everyone bury something in the middle of the batter—a dollop of jam, three or four mini-marshmallows, or chocolate squares are great.
- Cover the hidden treasure with more batter and bake.
- Since no one will be able to tell from the outside or remember whose is whose, everyone will be surprised when he or she discovers the hidden treasure buried in each cupcake.

PIGGIES IN BLANKETS
- Cut up gluten-free hot dogs, cooked sausage, or chunks of deli meat, or cheese (thickly sliced).
- Prepare gluten-free pizza crust or bread dough mix.
- Preheat the oven (according to the instructions on the package) and line baking sheets with parchment paper or aluminum foil.
- Spread out sheets of plastic wrap and give each person a small scoop of dough. Have him or her press the hot dog or other choice of pig into the dough, using the plastic wrap to coax the dough to cover the top completely so the pig is hidden.

- Use the plastic wrap to deliver the pig and blankets to the baking sheet. Bake them for about 15 minutes.
- You won't need a lot of dough for each pig, but you'll have a lot of giggles. In fact, young kids will want to oink each time they finish making one of these.

PIZZA PARTY

- Make your own personal-size gluten-free pizza dough rounds or buy a commercial brand of individual gluten-free pizza crusts.
- Hold a shop-a-thon and let the kids pick out their own toppings at the supermarket. (Okay, limit the budget or the choices for this one could break the bank.)
- Throw a contest to see who has made the most creative pizza. Take pictures of everyone eating his or her pizza and put them on a Facebook page if this is allowed, or send them to a school website.

SUGAR COOKIE EXTRAVAGANZA

- Make up a batch of gluten-free cookie dough and divide it into bowls.
- Let everyone add his or her own smoosh-ins—nuts, candies, or cut-up fruit rollups. Then bake the cookies.

Stocking your pantry with safe brands of go-to items will make life easier when you need to pull off one of these quick food events or put a quick meal or snack together for hungry kids. For safe brands, see Resources, page 312.

House Rules

You'll want to establish a few guidelines that help fold a special diet into family life:

- Set limits: choices are negotiable; eating gluten is not.
- Don't overdramatize the diet. Yes, it's a big deal, but no one needs to know that except you.

- Let the child and his or her siblings know, in age-appropriate terms, that gluten is not good for Mary or Joey to eat. Be firm and consistent: Mary cannot eat gluten and it's everyone's job to help her stay safe.
- Avoid threats or showing disappointment if the child gets gluten-ed.
- Don't rush to judgment or accuse anyone of "poisoning" the gluten-free person.
- Fortunately, a slipup is usually not going to require that your child be rushed to the hospital.

Have a Game Plan

Okay, you've got ideas for your household, but what about all the other situations that your kid will encounter as he or she ventures out into the world? Think: substitution. The trick is to find food that is equally delicious and gluten-free. Then it isn't obvious that your child is eating gluten-free pizza when everyone else is eating regular pizza, or a gluten-free cupcake when the rest of the group is eating cupcakes.

No parents want their children to feel different or left out. Kids say, just give them something. *They don't want to have nothing to eat.*

Be positive; be proactive:

- Find fun gluten-free treats that everyone can enjoy.
- Make up a list of school lunches, quick meals, and sports/travel snacks. (This may be a bunch of notes you keep in the glove compartment of the car or a formal list you tape to the fridge and share with sitters, grandparents, and the rest of the family.)
- Download lists of safe Halloween candies and Easter and Christmas treats, available on many websites. (Make a game of sorting candies collected during holidays. And keep some extra treats as backup in case that Halloween take didn't net the stash you hoped.)
- Educate caregivers, sitters, grandparents, and teachers (see page 236).
- Remind teachers frequently to let you know when treats will be served in the classroom so you can provide something for your child.
- Alert coaches, too, so you can discuss team parties and road stops after games.

Do-Ahead Checklist

You can't imagine all the ways that the GFD will seep into your child's activities. Whether it's playdates for youngsters, sleepovers for your teens, or other kid-centric events, use this list as a starting point to help you plan ahead.

- Car Stock. Keep a stash in the car—snack bars, dried fruit and nuts, individually wrapped cookies, and small bags of GF pretzels. Let all the kids share or keep this stash handy so the gluten-free child can select something when his siblings are eating snacks on the way to soccer practice or on a road trip. (You'll rely on this bag of treats more often than you know.)
- Parties. Make batches of cupcakes and sugar cookies. Wrap individually and freeze. Frost and decorate (with your child's help) to take to a schoolmate's birthday party, sports event, classroom parties, church events, or sleepover.
- Pizza Everything. Make up and freeze personal pizzas or parbake the crusts, or stash commercial gluten-free pizza crusts so these are ready for pizza parties.
- Sleepovers and Playdates. Keep GF hamburger and hot-dog rolls on hand. Talk to a host ahead and ask that a hamburger or hot dog be set aside for your child. (Check hot-dog brands to make sure they are safe.)

Commercial brands are available for nearly all gluten-free options. Although some are not as tasty as homemade versions, the convenience of having them on hand can be a godsend for busy parents.

Pre-K and Kindergarten

Finger paints, glue, paste, Play-Doh, face paints, papier-mâché, and even modeling clay are key elements in any young child's programs. But *everything* goes in the mouth, when it comes to little children and many brands contain wheat. It can be pretty hard to keep little fingers out of the mouth or prevent children from sampling the clay. And who doesn't love smearing finger paints all over the table and chairs?

In play groups, you'll be able to monitor your child's activity closely and provide safe alternatives, but it's harder when he or she enters preschool and kindergarten or has kid-only playdates.

Research the ingredients in the craft supplies used by the school and ask the staff to bring in safe equivalents. (There are many, including Mama K's Play Clay at mama-ks.com.) Also, remind teachers and aides to clean surfaces and wash sponges. And everyone should wash his or her hands after these activities to prevent your child from coming in contact with residual gluten. (They all should anyway.)

Some parents require their child to wear a surgical-type mask over the mouth while they participate in these activities as a reminder not to put fingers in the mouth. (I offer this as a suggestion, but frankly, it's not something I could ever do to my child.)

Snacks, too, need to be carefully monitored. You will provide safe alternatives, of course, but little kids are messy and surfaces and hands should be cleaned up after snacks, too. If teachers need more information, refer them to americanceliac.org, where they can download information under "Healthcare Professionals/School Nutrition" and the section called "For Families." (For more information, see "School Lunch" on page 238.)

Explaining the Gluten-free Diet to Babysitters and Grandparents

I put these in the same category as both are frequent visitors to your home and inherently care about your children. Too much information can overwhelm them but they need to understand that this diet is important to your child's health. Plus, no one wants to be cleaning up vomit or diarrhea on his or her watch.

Label all your child's foods with stickers or colors that everyone has agreed to. (We talked about that on page 152.) Set them in a separate cupboard or place if possible. Stock prepackaged gluten-free options (bonus—they are already labeled).

Designate a gluten-free toaster, jelly, peanut butter, and butter dish.

If you are leaving someone else in charge for a day, overnight, or a week, make a list of meals and snacks that are safe and put that list someplace where everyone can see it. Indicate where the foods are located (refrigerator or freezer or cupboard). Here's another reason one kid's special diet is a family affair. In your absence, the other siblings can help prevent diet mishaps. Keep things simple. Unless grandparents or babysitters are very familiar with this diet, it's easier not to have to explain separate pots for pasta or cross-contamination with cutting boards.

Going to Grandma's and other sleepovers can be stressful times when you add a GFD to the equation. But you don't want your child to miss out on these adventures. They are part of growing up. So fortify everyone with a few handy tips, and, again, keep the choices and instructions as simple as possible. Grandparents might keep a supply of food on hand that Tommy or Abby can have. Stocking gluten-free frozen pizza, chicken nuggets, cereal, bread, cookies, and a clean toaster might be all it takes. If the child is going to a babysitter's or friend's house for a sleepover, leave the toaster at home, but have the child pack some of the food choices on page 235 in his or her backpack. Remind the parent at a sleepover or the babysitter to remove the items and store them appropriately. For sleepovers, call the parents and alert them to what your child is bringing or ask what they plan to serve so you can provide the gluten-free versions. Go over a quick safety checklist to cut down on cross-contamination—don't share knives or butter or cutting boards, for example.

Label systems are available through kfk-enjoy.com and kidcals.com.

Sharing Custody

Who gets custody of a child's special diet when the marriage dissolves? No one is off the hook for this one. I've heard of situations where the gluten-free kid eats gluten-free with one parent, while the other parent ignores the diet. That's just plain unfair. It might even be grounds for a loss of visitation rights. But let's not go there.

Instead, both parents must take charge and be on the same page about this diet. I don't care if you need a mediator to help you. Just do it.

Incorporate the diet into all the preparations for switching homes. When the child is young, designate a travel case that is packed with favorite gluten-free foods. And give the child coupons and a list of safe, kid-friendly restaurants, too. The resources can be passed back and forth. Buy a designated gluten-free toaster for both homes, too.

As your child grows, he or she can take more responsibility and participate in more of the choices. He or she might even take charge of meal planning or do some of the baking.

Note: You may have negotiated your divorce, but your kid's health is nonnegotiable. Please, don't use it to get back at your ex.

School Lunch: Take It or Buy It (a 504 Plan)

We talked about lunch in Part 2, but it's a different game when your kid's at school. Many parents prefer to make their child's lunch every day so they know it is free of contamination and healthy and well balanced. (See more on lunch ideas on page 155.)

But you can also ask your school system to provide a gluten-free meal for your child without additional cost (other than the regular cost of school lunch).

The American Celiac Disease Alliance, an organization that advocates for patient needs, says students who must adhere to a medically prescribed diet may qualify for special dietary accommodations under the National School Lunch Program (NHLP). If your child attends a public school that participates in the NHLP, the school must (1) provide special meal accommodations; (2) the parent or guardian is not required to furnish those gluten-free products; and (3) foods served must be purchased by the school from commercial sources.

Even if your child attends a private school that provides lunches to its students, it, too, must make accommodations under the Americans with Disabilities Act.

Bringing in gluten-free food and asking the cafeteria staff to serve it might violate the local health code. But packing a lunch for your child is still an option. You, your child, and the school will need to find a solution that is most comfortable for the child and still keeps him or her safe.

You can also file a 504 plan (a documented disability) with your school system. This requires a bit of paperwork, lots of documentation (e.g., letters from your child's physician), and meetings with key school officials. In addition to a lunch program, it includes a classroom management plan. A 504 plan for a young child might include a request to notify the parent before any food is used in the classroom; that hands and tables be wiped carefully after a snack; and that the child wears a surgical mask when working with food materials, to remind him or her not to touch his mouth until the mask comes off.

American Celiac Disease Alliance, americanceliac.org, and National Foundation for Celiac Awareness, celiaccentral.org, have sample plans on their websites.

Sports Events

A swim meet, soccer tournament, or other sports event is often followed by a team meal at a fast-food or pizza place on the way home. This can get dicey for a child on a GFD.

Let the coach know about your child's diet and emphasize that this is a medical necessity. Work together to pick a place where gluten-free options are available. Wendy's, Red Robin, and Outback are always good options, where everyone likes the food and gluten-free choices are available.

Bullying

I had all kinds of clever titles for this section—Food Wars, Food Fights, Weaponized Peanuts. But in the end, I eliminated each one. There is nothing clever or funny about this subject. It breaks my heart that our kids often face the double whammy of living with a food sensitivity and being singled out as different in the classroom

In fact, a 2010 study in the journal *Annals of Allergy, Asthma & Immunology* reports that 35 percent of kids over age five with food allergies have been bullied or teased in school. It gets much harder when the kid has a life-threatening allergy such as to peanuts or nuts, as everyone in the classroom has to be reminded about the child's allergy every time there's a snack, a party, or a food project.

Sometimes the child is singled out and then bullied. Kids throw that food at the child or try to force him or her to eat it, to see what will happen. *Traumatic* only begins to describe the feeling of terror that these kids face every day.

Another study in the journal *Pediatrics* found that more than 30 percent of children have been harassed by their classmates because of their allergies, and that parents are only aware of it about half of the time.

The more frequent the bullying, the worse the child's quality of life, the study found. But just one instance of bullying took a toll on a kid's happiness. And when parents knew about these incidents, the child's quality of life improved.

Watch for changes in your child's behavior. Such signs as being withdrawn, not wanting to go to school, not wanting to bring a lunch, or all-around moodiness can be signals. Be proactive and address these issues with a school nurse or social worker, the teacher, and the child.

That said, kids with gluten issues are less likely to encounter this kind of bullying. No one needs to caution students to keep bread away from a student who can't have gluten and the food can look fairly normal. Kids learn to fake it by either not eating in front of peers or eating a salad or something else that everyone can eat.

That's not to say these kids don't feel different or excluded or feel the need to explain why their sandwich looks different or why they never take hot lunch. Fortunately, a gluten issue does not often reach the level where just having the food in the same area will cause the child to become sick. But it's horribly embarrassing if a child has an accident in his pants or throws up because he's eaten something containing gluten.

Some schools also require kids to sit at allergy-free tables, which is both a blessing and a curse. (I am certain my son would never have consented to sit at a separate table.) I understand that this is a safety precaution for the school. But it really does make the kids feel different.

It's up to the parents and the teachers to empower the kids to talk about their food sensitivities freely and in a positive way. I'm a big advocate of running a "This is just part of who I am" campaign early in the school year so that every kid gets to share something that is special and different about him or her. A project done in the interest of "getting to know you," lessens the opportunities to turn differences against each other.

The Emotional Toll of Two Diets:
Type 1 Diabetes and Celiac Disease

These two autoimmune diseases seem to share a common genetic link. Typically between 5 and 10 percent of people (usually kids) who are diagnosed with type 1 diabetes will also be diagnosed with celiac disease. Managing two diets and monitoring blood sugar and insulin injections can be overwhelming for parents and children.

Diabetes is usually diagnosed first. Physicians should screen their patients for celiac disease within a year of being diagnosed with diabetes. In any case, if the child's blood sugar is difficult to manage, that is often a signal to test for celiac disease even sooner. If the child tests positive for celiac disease, after a period of healing, the blood sugar issues will also improve.

Finding a dietitian who is knowledgeable on both diseases is essential in handling this combination of regimens as they need to be managed in tandem.

Bottom line: A strict gluten-free diet is essential in helping to manage the diabetes component. But it's not a panacea. Gluten-free processed food tends to be high in simple carbohydrates, which metabolize very quickly. Following a healthy diet that is high in vegetables, dairy, and lean protein with nutrient-dense carbohydrates is key. The latter includes whole-grain flours, such as amaranth, quinoa, sorghum, millet, gluten-free oats, and chickpea, as well as legumes and nuts.

A note about type 2 diabetes and celiac disease: Type 2 diabetes was primarily a condition that affects adults, but no longer. More children are being diagnosed with type 2 diabetes than ever before. The good news is that the incidence of type 2 diabetes, the kind associated most often with age, weight gain (body mass index) and metabolic syndrome, is actually significantly lower in people with celiac disease, according to a study in the May 2013 issue of *Gastroenterology*.[1]

Mikey's Story

"When I was told our son had type 1 diabetes (22 months of age), I quickly learned to read food labels and count the carbohydrates of everything that went into his mouth, as well as how foods high in fat and fiber and/or protein interacted with the absorption rates of the insulin that we had to inject into Mikey each day.

"After the diagnosis of celiac disease was added, food became even more of an issue. We had to give up most of our go-to foods and try to find replacements (gluten-free of course). I found that many gluten-free foods (that taste good) are much higher in carbohydrates (sugars), and fat making it more of a challenge to keep Mikey's blood sugar under control. The calories are often much higher, too—so finding great tasting food that is gluten-free and diabetes-friendly is not always easy.

"Our go-to snack when Mikey has activities is gluten-free crackers and cream cheese or peanut butter with no added fat and sugar. We also finally found a granola bar that he enjoys.

"It's always a juggling act. It's not only food . . . stress, illness, exercise, and even extreme weather can affect Mikey's blood sugar. His diet involves the entire family. And that helps. We've always all participated in this and I think that helps to keep his attitude bright and sunny despite the fact that he has a lot more to worry about than the average teenager."

—OKSANA CHARLA, MOTHER OF MIKEY, AGE 15

Depression and Diet

Kids with both celiac disease and type 1 diabetes are more apt to experience depression. While it may be normal, it's hardly a welcome addition to the juggling act of managing two diagnoses.

Aside from simply coping with being different, bullying at school can also be a factor in mood changes and depression. A school social worker or psychologist can be a helpful ally in managing the emotional component. I've included a few ideas to help your child have a positive experience coping with a special diet. You'll probably have a few of your own to add. (See "Kids and the GFD" and "Bullying," pages 226 and 239.)

Teenagers: Peer Versus Parent

Pleasing teenagers can be difficult—okay, impossible. Add the challenge of a gluten-free diet, and it can be a daunting task. But teens are old enough to understand the consequences of eating gluten.

Let teens take charge of the diet and let them be the ones to contact hosts about parties. Remind them that it's their body and their health and that soon they will be off to college, where they will be fully responsible for the diet.

Let them shop for their own food and make it. Teens will eat what they make, plus they'll learn about the diet at the same time. Remind your teen that a healthy body means that he or she will look and feel better (shiny hair, bright eyes, clearer skin, more energy), and perform better in class and sports. Besides, no one wants to miss out on the high school prom or college homecoming weekend because of feeling crappy. Ultimately they have to live with the consequences of their actions. (Isn't that the message anyway?)

As for the "anti's"—drugs and smoking—you'll be adding gluten to the list. Have that talk in private before your teen goes out for the evening. Ask him or her, "How will you handle eating out tonight?"

Romancing the Gluten-Honeymoon Period

The teenage years are when kids feel the most invincible. There's evidence that some teens with celiac disease may be asymptomatic when they are entering puberty (ages ten to fifteen); that is, when they cheat, they don't feel the effects. Nevertheless, damage is still occurring. This used to be called the honeymoon period and goes back to the days when we believed that celiac was a childhood disease and that kids outgrew it. Gluten was reintroduced just about the time that these kids were hitting puberty. Symptoms and rediagnosis did not take place until later in life, often triggered by pregnancy, illness, or a life stress. There's no such thing as "outgrowing" celiac disease, so the term is not used much anymore, but teenagers are still rebellious and their being asymptomatic may lead to cheating on the GFD.

Is it rebellion against the diet or against parental authority? It's difficult to separate the two. Growing up is all about taking control over one's own life and the reasons for being on a gluten-free diet are not something teens can control. Keep the dialogue going and remind your teens they are the only ones hurt when they cheat.

What to Do When Your Kid Wants to Cheat

My son was eleven when he announced that he was going to eat an egg roll someone brought to our New Year's Eve party. "Go ahead. It's your body," I said, never thinking he would eat it. To my horror, he did. "Well," I thought. "I hope he gets good and sick." But I didn't say a word. He told me later that he never had a reaction. I'm not so sure. I don't think he ever knowingly cheated again.

At age twelve, he took his lunch to school, but ordered French fries every day. Soon he started having celiac symptoms again. After visiting the school, I discovered the fries were coated with wheat. He stopped eating them as soon as I mentioned it. If he had a honeymoon period, it was a short-lived romance. Lesson learned.

Not every parent will have this exact experience (or response!), but I bet at some point you'll have resistance from a kid who just wants to be "normal"—and/or test the boundaries. So what are you supposed to do? Of course, if your child gets symptoms when he or she cheats, that can be motivation enough to stick to the diet.

If a child is asymptomatic, it's worth the extra reminder that damage is still going on even without symptoms: Like a car, you might say, you perform better when you are tuned up and in tip-top shape. You'll feel and look your best, do well in school and sports, and grow to your fullest height. (If nothing else resonates, the last point will.)

Cheating is serious business. Discuss the seriousness of celiac disease, but stay upbeat. *Don't reprimand or punish your kid for cheating or talking about it.* No one wins when you fight over gluten.

My son was one of the original campers at Camp Celiac (see page 246). At a gathering of his camp friends, I asked the question, "What do you do when you want to cheat?" They began to cackle. They enjoyed the vicarious thrill of imagining they were eating a slice of chocolate cake. But, to my surprise, not one of the teens confessed to cheating—not even once.

Yes, teens are fickle creatures, but ultimately they want to do what's best for them. Those hundreds of conversations you had when you felt as if you were talking to a brick wall—well, some of them sink in. So, when you have that talk about cheating, remind your teen that there are decadent, safe options that let him or her enjoy the same kinds of foods as what friends are eating—just prepared gluten-free. Think: buffalo wings, lasagne (recipe on page 185), tacos, nachos, fajitas, chocolate chip cookies (recipe on page 180), brownies, ice cream, and hot fudge.

What do you think gluten-free teens do when they go out with their friends, to look normal and avoid cheating? Here's what this group from Camp Celiac said:

- Eat first and go for the company.
- Encourage friends to go someplace that has gluten-free pizza.
- Order a root beer float.
- Have a Coke and chips.
- Order a hamburger on a lettuce wrap and tell them, "I'm dieting."
- Pick a gluten-free-friendly restaurant.

One more reminder: Teens are *not* apt to bring their own food to a restaurant or house party. Let them figure out the most comfortable way to handle each situation. Be there to support and discuss the options.

Gluten-free Camp

Gluten-free camps, both day and overnight experiences, are available all over the country. They offer empowering and enriching experience for both young kids and teens. Some are private camps and others are operated by celiac patient support groups. A lot of mainstream camps are getting an accreditation to serve gluten-free meals for celiac campers, too.

Gut Reaction: Cheating—Not Just for Kids

Years ago three gluten-free friends went out for dinner at a nice restaurant in Washington, DC. The chef-owner promised to cook us a gluten-free meal. As we chortled and moaned over the panoply of flavors, the marriage of fresh herbs, and the parade of courses, we started talking gluten-free.

"What do you do when you want to cheat?" someone asked. "I sniff the bread in the bread basket," said one. "I lick the frosting off éclairs," confessed another. "I chew and spit," I responded. "Ewww," they screamed as if no one else was in the restaurant. "Well, I don't do it anymore. But I used to before I knew how chancy it was," I confessed.

At that, someone repeated, "Chew and spit," and we practically split a gluten-free gut laughing. Note: Anytime gluten meets the mouth, it's inevitable that some of it will be ingested. (Remember the story about the person who got sick from her toothpaste, page 87?) Don't take a chance.

Start by checking the local support group websites and the Celiac Listserv for information, and sign up early. Spaces fill up quickly. Wherever you live, consider giving your child a camp experience. "The bond is magical—binding kids who are like themselves without talking about it," says Lisa Walton, codirector, Camp Celiac, North Scituate, Rhode Island.

Camp binds kids together. "They feel safe and don't worry about diet so they can enjoy other events," she says.

One camper describes it this way: "You don't meet friends at camp, you meet your 'family.' We have grown up together, and will always be there for each other no matter how far the distance may be. Camp isn't just a week for us, it's a lifetime."

Young Adults: College Bound and Gluten-free

I know I have said more than once: don't let your diet define you. And don't pick a college based on whether it can accommodate the GFD.

Nevertheless, these are four important years of your child's life. He or she will be forging new friendships, studying hard, playing even harder (hmm). You want him or her to have a great college experience, one that makes your child feel included not excluded from activities. After all, who wants to feel crappy and tired all the time or worried about getting sick in front of friends (or anytime)? So, just like academic programs, makeup of the student body, location, the football team, and whether the girls or guys are hot, diet is an important part of the checklist when you and your nearly high-school-graduate look at college.

My son attended Columbia University in New York City at just about the time that gluten-free was becoming trendy. We contacted the manager of food service and the dietitian beforehand. We met with the chef, who went through the entire menu with us. "We have kosher and vegan offerings. I don't see why we couldn't do gluten-free as well," he said. He stocked GF bagels and bread and cereal in a designated location and set up a separate toaster for Jeremy and four others who wanted the gluten-free option. He told Jeremy to call anytime if he had questions about the menu.

We asked housing to give him a room on a floor with a kitchen and asked permission for him to have a refrigerator in his room.

As it turns out, the meal plan was based on points and Jeremy used his to order an omelet and a couple of GF bagels for brunch every day. Sometimes he had a salad later in the day. The rest of the time, he cooked in the dorm or ordered take-out from local eateries that had a gluten-free menu.

He never talked to the chef again! So, while I followed my own best advice about the college experience, my son did not. But read "Lindsey's Story," page 250 or Rob's story, below, to learn the lengths that a college will go to accommodate their gluten-free students.

In talking to experts on this subject, I discovered about half of college students (more men than women) are shy about dealing with their diet on campus.

My friend Rob Landolphi confirmed that he sees that avoidance preference at his campus, too. Rob is the manager of culinary development at the University of Connecticut at the Storrs Campus and instituted a gluten-free dining option in all the dining facilities beginning in 2002. Rob, whose wife and middle son have celiac disease, is also the author of three gluten-free cookbooks. He is part of a team of five who meet with every prospective student who requests the gluten-free dining option at the University of Connecticut. They talk about all the products and the ingredients and the protocol for serving gluten-free meals in the eight facilities.

The goal is to put students at ease—to make them feel included and comfortable, and make it possible to eat with their friends. A doctor's note is not required. There is no extra fee for gluten-free dining options and the food is not served in a separate allergen-free room. UCONN does not want to segregate the students with special diets. However, there is a gluten-free zone where students can help themselves to cereals, toasters, and a refrigerator stocked with gluten-free foods.

If students are shy, they don't have to speak to anyone. Every single dish is labeled for the eight top food allergens plus gluten. But they will have to ask if they want gluten-free pasta and marinara sauce, or cold cuts. To avoid cross-contamination, these are stored away from the regular food service line.

Rob says that 15 to 20 percent of the total food prepared each day is gluten-free, including at least two entrée options and the salad bar.

The campus food service tries to incorporate gluten-free ingredients in as many preparations as possible. For instance, they use ground Rice Chex in vegan burgers and for breading.

"We see a lot of food service manufacturers switching to gluten-free ingredients. Many of our salad dressings, stir-fry sauces, taco shells, nacho chips, and cold cuts already say 'gluten-free' on the label. It makes our life much easier," says Rob.

Here are some of Rob's best tips for prepping for a gluten-free life, college-style:

When you are looking at colleges . . .

- Contact Dining Services or Residential Life directly. (The name of the office will vary from college to college.)
- Ask how it handles gluten-free diets.
- Ask to set up a tour of the dining hall and the kitchen.
- If the staff's guard goes up or if they seem hesitant, be wary.

- If you are shown the kitchen and served a gluten-free lunch, that should put your mind at ease.
- Ask whether the college offers gluten-free foods in all the dining facilities. If not, find out how far the gluten-free dining hall is from your dorm and the buildings where you will be taking most of your classes.
- Check the hours of operations.
- Find out whether gluten-free food is prepared in a designated area.
- Does the college label all the food so it's not necessary to locate a chef each time you eat in the dining hall?
- Does the dining hall have a gluten-free zone?
- Can you eat in the same area as your friends or is gluten-free food served only in a separate dining room?
- What gluten-free brands are used? Is the staff willing to bring in other brands?
- What happens if you don't like the option for that day? Can you order something else?
- Can you call ahead and order food?
- Is there a website where you can find out the options for the day?
- Does the gluten-free option cost more money or is it included in your meal plan? (It should be included.)
- What restaurants near campus have gluten-free choices? Do they deliver? (This will be useful for times when your friends are ordering out and you don't want to be left out.)
- Ask to speak with a student who has been taking the gluten-free option. Chances are, at least one or two have offered to serve as a resource.

If the answers to any of these questions are not to your liking, it's not necessarily a deal breaker. You might need to contact housing to request a dorm room near a kitchen area and permission to have small appliances.

These handy appliances will make you feel more at home in a college dorm room:

- Mini refrigerator
- Rice cooker

- Microwave oven
- Hot pot (to heat soup, chili, and water for dehydrated meals and beverages)

Note: Toasters, tabletop grills, hot plates, toaster ovens, and griddles are not allowed.

Well Fed, Well Schooled: Lindsey's Story

Lindsey Schnitt is one person who wasn't shy when it came to managing her gluten-free diet in college. A recent graduate of Penn State, Lindsey bought her own food the first year of college and brought it to the kitchen. As she got to know the chef, he told her to call ahead and he would prepare whatever she wanted. When she moved to another part of campus, food service bought the food and stocked it for her. The staff set up a separate fryer, prepared gluten-free soups, and made just about every option available to her.

"We got so used to working together. After a while, the chef would say he thought I should eat more vegetables and he would add them for me."

She became well known. The head of food service invited her to give a presentation to the trustees. Following her presentation, gluten-free became a full-fledged option in food service throughout the campus. Foods are labeled so students with gluten and other food sensitivities can navigate the dining hall with their friends.

"My success at school was based on being well fed. If finding safe food was tough, I'm sure I would have had a different outcome. You'd think you would get lost in such a big school, but not at all," says Schnitt.

A Case for Americans with Disabilities:
What Happens When a University Fails?

It was just the opposite at Lesley University in Cambridge, Massachusetts, where students needing a gluten-free diet recently won a settlement after a complaint was filed claiming the university was falling short of the Americans with Disabilities Act requirements. The basis of the complaint was that the university did not offer additional gluten-free food options requested by students. An agreement was reached in December 2012. As a result, Lesley is now offering a broad selection of gluten-free choices on campus.

"If the university was meeting student needs, it wouldn't need to come to this. A lot of universities today are already offering gluten-free options. When it comes right down to it, we are already accommodating nut-free and vegan diets. It seems funny that colleges wouldn't accommodate this one group," says Rob Landolphi.

Making the Grade: Top Gluten-free-Friendly Schools

At udisglutenfree.com, students chose their Top Gluten Free Accommodating College Campuses, evaluating them for a list of services ranging from separate dining areas to separate gluten-free stations to detailed labeling and staff training.

But don't worry if your school isn't included in this slightly biased list. Dozens more are listed by current and former students at glutenfreetravelsite.com (go to "gluten-free college reviews") and at celiac.com. A list of GFF colleges and universities can be found in Resources, page 310.

Privacy and Parents

As a result of the Health Insurance Portability and Accountability Act (HIPAA), parents cannot talk to the health center staff without their child's permission (because he or she is over 18). Not only can you not check on your children's mental and physical health through the college health service, but if students need medicines that are prescribed through the college infirmary or over the counter, they are on their own to verify that these are gluten-free. As they are big boys and girls and you've taught them well, this should not be a difficult class to pass; nevertheless, you may want to have a chat with your kids to make sure they know that, to a certain extent, at college their health really is their own responsibility.

Resources for College-Bound Kids

Celiaccentral.org, the official site of the National Foundation for Celiac Awareness (NFCA), produces helpful material on planning for college. Check out its online publications *Gluten-free Guide to College Living*; *Celiacs and College: Tips for Parents and Prospective Students*; and *Gluten Free Guide to College*.

A Rite of GF Passage:
Playing Beer Pong Without Beer

Beer Pong is as much a college requirement as freshman English. Flunk it and you might become a social outcast. The pressure is on. However, how do you play Beer Pong when you can't drink beer? Sure, gluten-free beer is available. But it's pricey. Even if your bank account is flush, who wants to waste expensive beer on a drinking game? Plus, some gluten-free beer is not as tasty as the barley hop–based stuff. The last thing you want is for your friends to criticize your taste in beer.

Kids who are gluten-free and entering college can use finesse to gracefully blend their diet with college drinking games.

If you're not familiar with Beer Pong, the premise is simple:

Plastic cups filled with beer are lined up, bowling pin fashion, on each end of a long table, preferably an old Ping-Pong table or a piece of plywood, and not someone's dining room table. Each cup is filled halfway with beer. Each team stands behind its rows of beer-filled glasses with two Ping-Pong balls. The object is to get the ball into one of the cups on the opponents' side. If successful, the opponent has to drink the beer and removes the cup. The winner is the team that sunk all the balls in the opponents' cups. The losing team has drunk the most beer. It seems like nobody really loses, unless you can't drink regular beer. However, this game can be played with other beverages. Most kids who can't drink beer, or don't like the taste, use water and keep a beverage of their choice on the side.

My friend Kelsey Haggett prefers water instead of beer. "This way everyone can keep their own drink and sip from it while they play. It's a lot more sanitary, too," says the recent college graduate who was diagnosed with celiac disease during her freshman year.

My son prefers to stand on the sidelines, watch others play, and make small talk. He and Kelsey are both up front about the fact that they can't drink regular beer. If the other players act like jerks, they just move on to another social event. After some practice, your child will figure out the most comfortable strategy. And, hey, not everyone takes calculus and no one says you have to play Beer Pong. Whether it's Beer Pong or any other activity that involves unsafe food (or drink), these are good strategies to employ.

Adults: Eating with the Enemy

House Parties: Guest Who's Coming to Dinner

Gut Reaction: Grill the Host or Get Skewered

A friend from Chicago was visiting friends in Boston and invited me to meet him for dinner. Tom was not a good friend, more of a business acquaintance, someone I knew from the gluten-free trade show circuit. He has a witty sense of humor that makes him great company, but as it turns out, not the best person to trust with the seriousness of a gluten-free diet.

As our "date" grew closer, the plans expanded to include an invitation to dinner at his college roommate's house in a Boston suburb. "Keith is making his famous veal dish and wants us to join them," said Tom. It seemed chancy—the casual friend of a casual acquaintance. Too many degrees of separation for me. But against my better judgment, I accepted. I stuffed a gluten-free roll in my purse, just in case.

"Does he know about my diet?" I asked. I knew that Tom was pretty knowledgeable, being that he marketed a gluten-free product line.

"He says, no worries. We have plenty of gluten," Tom joked. The humor gave me false hope. I assumed that meant he had explained the details and we were good. So I made the two-hour journey from Connecticut to join them.

We met at a coffeehouse on Beacon Hill. It was February and the entire Northeast was coated in a thick layer of ice. As we walked back to the car, Tom slipped and landed on his right arm, shattering two bones.

We drove to his friend's house by way of an emergency room, calling to say we'd be late. By the time the cast was applied and painkillers

▶

▼

administered, it was nearly eight o'clock. Tom's humor had vanished and he was, understandably, wallowing in self pity. Me, too. But mine was from hunger pains.

When we arrived, dinner was already being served and we were quickly escorted to the table. A couple I did not know was waiting, two drinks and plates of appetizers under their belts. "Let's eat," said Keith's wife. The icebreaker moments were past, a time where I might have said, "Hi. I'm Beth and I have celiac disease."

As we settled into our seats in their formal dining room, the hostess placed a china plate in front of each of us. "It's Keith's famous Wiener Schnitzel and Spatzle," she announced. "His grandmother's recipe."

I looked down at a heavily breaded veal cutlet swimming in brown gravy, egg noodles diving under more pools of gravy, and green beans drowning in another pool of flour-laden brown liquid. There was no salad!

I looked around desperately. Tom, well stewed on painkillers and two Scotches, was oblivious. I could not find an ally nor could I pretend to eat.

What's more, my purse and gluten-free roll were in the living room. I was too embarrassed to retrieve it and eat in front of this group.

I could leave you in suspense and leave me at the table in one of the most embarrassing moments of my life.

I would like to say there is a teaching moment here, but I think of this experience as more of the perfect gluten-free storm, a time for which all the stockpiling in the world could not help.

I've learned to be a bit more assertive since that evening and directly contact the folks who wield the knives, leaving less room for miscommunication and embarrassing moments. I give the hosts the opportunity to uninvite me if they think it is too difficult to accommodate my diet. I'm happy to tell you no one has ever accepted an uninvitation opportunity. But that introduction affords me the chance to grab their attention and make them realize my diet is a serious matter. Then I am able to discuss the menu and find places where I can contribute. It also gives fair warning in case I cannot partake, saving face for both parties.

▶

> ▼
>
> In this instance, the hostess finally noticed I was not eating. "I'm afraid I can't," I confessed, smiling awkwardly behind a crimson face. She gathered me and my plate and together we found a few green beans that had not been adulterated in schnitzel juice and a couple of leftover slices of cheese.
>
> We both learned something that night. Tom will likely never again wear loafers to Boston in February. And I will never rely on a third person to convey my dietary needs.

How to Tell a Host About Your Diet

Gluten-ed by proxy. When you relax your dietary vigilance and trust that the person preparing your food knows the GFD as well as you do, you risk being gluten-ed by proxy. We all do it. Perhaps we assume too much, communicate too little, or the gluten-free radar is down because we are tired of this process. Whatever the reason, that false sense of security can spell trouble.

Being invited to dinner at someone's home arguably has the most potential for creating an awkward situation. You are on someone else's turf and at the mercy of that person's adaptability. When you have to ask a bunch of questions about what's being served and how things are made (i.e., grill the host), it's easy to move out of your comfort zone.

Although I am seldom at a loss for words, invitations to people's homes often leave me speechless and less than assertive about my diet. Because these are so personal, I find eating at someone's home is more uncomfortable than eating in a restaurant. Find your inner strength and put awkwardness aside, or suffer the consequences and get gluten-ed by proxy.

Here are some basic tips to help you break the ice:

Cut Out the Middle Man

Don't count on someone else to convey your dietary needs to a host. Get the phone number or e-mail address for the host and say you are looking forward to coming for dinner but need to tell him or her about your diet.

Offer to bring something. "I'd like to make a special dish to go with your meal. Will this fit with the menu you are planning?"

Your host will be grateful for your thoughtful offer. And even if the menu is already planned, it's a great segue into talking about your diet, which dishes could be a problem, and which might be safe with a tiny tweak.

When it's awkward or you're just too shy, bring a gluten-free dessert or an antipasto platter. Like a bottle of wine or a box of chocolates, these are nice hostess gifts without being intrusive. No guarantee that your host will serve them, however. But if nothing else is safe to eat, it's okay to suggest putting out the item you brought.

First time at the boss's house or a business get-together. A cake or an edible fruit bouquet is always welcome and neutral. And it doesn't imply a culinary takeover. But it won't be enough for a meal. Consider eating something at home and pack a gluten-free roll or crackers you can have with cheese. Isn't there's always a cheese platter?!

Be a Snoop

All your preparty diligence cannot prevent surprises. Many people are simply not aware of all the hidden ingredients in packaged foods.

Whether you've had the "talk" with your host or not, arrive early to help. That gives you a chance to survey the kitchen for gluten traps, such as croutons or crunchy salad toppings (that contain wheat). Usually a telltale package is still around. Pick it up and casually glance at the label: "This looks interesting. Oh dear, I see that it has wheat." This gives you a chance to ask whether the topping or croutons or other gluteny ingredient could be served on the side.

Take Stock of Your Approach

When you speak to the host about your diet, how do you come across?

- Don't whine. Too much negative information can overwhelm your host.
- Be confident. "Together I know we can create something safe."
- Be appreciative of a lovely dinner invitation.

- Give the host an out. "I have a medically prescribed gluten-free diet and if it's too difficult, we can join you for coffee and dessert." (No one uninvites a guest.)
- Offer to go out to a restaurant that has a gluten-free menu.
- If you are the only one(s) invited, suggest that the host come to your house. (You can take more control this way.)

Working Together to Build a Safe Meal
If your host-to-be is willing, here are some great suggestions to build a meal together. First of all, start with a stripped-down menu:

- Plain baked potato or plain rice
- Naked meat or fish (no marinade, crumb coating, or flour)
- Salad without dressing, croutons, or crunchy toppings
- Ice cream or fruit for dessert

If the host is receptive, add onto the basics:

- Ask what's in the marinade. Add it back if safe or suggest one that is.
- Ask about the salad dressing. Add that back if it's okay.
- If the host is making rice, inquire about preparation, brand of chicken broth, and such. Have the rice if it's okay.
- Skip dessert. Actually, don't skip it! Ask whether ice cream or fruit is part of the dessert and have one of those.

If the host seems resistant to making alterations, put on your Take-Charge hat:

- Offer to bring a main-course dish that you know is safe; in fact, *insist* (nicely).
- Make gluten-free brownies or cookies or buy a frozen variety.
- Throw in a pint of gluten-free sorbet or ice cream and chocolate syrup.
- Bring a stash of bread and crackers.
- Be self-sufficient but not pushy.

See "GF Foods You Can Serve to Your Fanciest Company" on page 159 and recipes are on pages 170–191.

Be Thankful for Buffets and Potlucks

Often, you can easily contribute a hearty (and safe) dish to the mix—a salad with protein, a gluten-free pasta salad, risotto with meat, lasagne, or a vegetable dish are all good choices to bring. Be first in line. Or remove a portion and set it aside before serving spoons comingle and the food gets contaminated. I like to set my plate on top of the refrigerator if possible, so it's out of the way.

Grill Meat, Not People

Ask a host to grill your burger or plain piece of meat first before hamburger buns and meats with marinade come in contact with the grid. But first, make sure the grill has been heated and scraped so the grid is free of any gluten remnants. Or set a sheet of aluminum foil on top of the grid and poke holes in it so juices can drain and some of that great smoky flavor seeps into you food.

Make It a Picnic for You

Floppy sunhats and big sunglasses are perfect picnic garb. So are those colorful Tupperware containers with matching, sealable lids. But dishes, like visitors, come and go at a picnic and it's not clear who brought them, let alone what's in them. Unless the organizer asks people to identify the ingredients in each dish (which is not a bad idea), you're really putting your diet at risk if you dig in just because the ingredients look safe. Bring something you like and spoon out a portion to put aside. Grill a burger or chicken or hot dog that you know is safe, taking care to scrape the grill first. Stand guard while your food is cooking, lest someone tries to warm a roll next to your food.

Icebreakers for a Party

Good things about being diagnosed with celiac disease:

- **You won't find us in the Cheetos and Cheez Whiz sections.**

We can't eat most of the processed foods.

- **The incidence of breast cancers is lower in women with celiac disease.**

There is some evidence it might also be lower in women with gluten sensitivity, although the science is newer for this category.

A study in the *British Medical Journal* found the rate of breast cancer in celiac women about 40 percent lower than in the general population. It may be because women with celiac disease tend to get their period later, enter menopause earlier, and generally have lower fertility levels.

- **The rate of cardiovascular disease, metabolic syndrome, and type 2 diabetes is lower in people with celiac disease.**

This came out in a paper introduced at Digestive Disease Week, May 2013 and printed in May 2013 issue of *Gastroenterology*. In this paper, the researchers from Beth Israel Deaconess Medical Center (BIDMC) noted that celiac patients studied had lower body mass index and tend to smoke less.[2]

- **We eat healthier diets with more natural, minimally processed foods and foods with fewer additives.**

That's a no-brainer. The fewer ingredients, the safer the products for our diet. And most vegetables, fruits, meats, and dairy are gluten-free.

- **We eat better when we go to restaurants.**

How many gluten-free desserts do you see on the menu? And how many celiac or gluten-sensitive folks do you see grazing at the China Buffet?

- **We tend to smoke less.[3]**

Perhaps being on a GFD makes us more aware of our overall health.

13

Friendship, Dating, Love & Sex

A Glass Half-Full

Okay, I understand how embarrassing it can be to wear the wrong attire to a dance or pose for a photo sporting a long strand of spinach between your teeth. Those are things that you could change if you only knew. But eating gluten-free? It shouldn't be awkward. It's part of you, something you can't change. And it's about your health, for goodness' sake. If you look at the proverbial glass as half-full instead of half-empty, there's something special about a special diet. Socially, it can be an icebreaker (see topics on page 258). At the same time, it's an opportunity to make others aware that we don't all eat alike. Besides, these days, nearly everyone knows somebody who is on a gluten-free diet. It's totally fashionable. You are in style, no matter what you wear.

Friends Don't Let Friends Eat Gluten

If this regimen was just about the food, it wouldn't be such a big deal. We could hide in a closet, eat enough safe, gluten-free food to sustain us, then rejoin the world, no stigma attached. But food permeates every part of our lives. That's why this is the "lifestyle" section—where to eat, how to explain the diet, who to trust when you are feeling gluten-ed.

People respect a person for taking good care of him- or herself. So, work to create positive energy about yourself and your diet and how to attract people who are the same way.

Your mission, which I hope you will accept, is to avoid caustic relatives and friends who think this gluten thing is all in your head or that it's just a passing fad. (We all know one or two.) When you feel the negative energy flowing into your life, nix the downers. These people don't have your best interest at heart.

If you are gluten-free by choice, you might have an even tougher time convincing friends you do not want to eat gluten. You are part of a huge trend and there is always someone who thinks he or she know more than you do about trends. Fortitude, my friend. But remember that if you make an argument for why you have chosen to be gluten-free and then devour a big slice of regular pizza, your reasoning may have lost its teeth.

Gut Reaction:
Love Means Never Having to Eat Gluten

"Help! I'm losing all my friends! They think I'm strange because of this crazy gluten-free diet," wailed a young woman who contacted me after being diagnosed with celiac disease. *Awkward* and *embarrassing* were two words she repeated often.

A vague feeling of disquiet rumbled in my gut. This time it wasn't gluten. I was recalling my own battles with diet and friends.

As a young adult, I grappled with my own gluten-denial. "Just a little bit won't hurt me," I thought. When I went out with friends or on a date, I made certain things I ordered were not breaded or dusted with flour, but if a sauce looked clear, I ate it. Chinese restaurants were the worst. I loved Chinese food and ate it regularly although I knew most of the sauces contained wheat. (Don't *ever* do that, please!) For years I suffered from low-grade flulike symptoms but refused to consider they might be related to my gluten transgressions.

▶

I felt healthy when I ate stir-fry at home and tried to fool myself into believing that all Chinese food must be that safe. I taught Chinese cooking and used the traditional wheat-laden sauces. At the end of each class, I joined my hungry students in the feast we had prepared.

One day, the years of neglecting my health caught up with me.

While frantically double-parking to pick up a last-minute gift, I slammed my car door on my middle finger. The doctor at a nearby emergency room stitched my finger and bound it in an oh-so-attractive bracket bandage.

The bandaged digit garnered a good amount of sympathy, especially among my Chinese cooking students, one of whom was also a physician at that emergency room.

He made a house call and invited me to dinner at a Chinese restaurant. Despite the problematic menu, I did not say no.

At Peking Gourmet, I juggled a fork around my injured middle finger, flashing an obscene gesture as I ate. But truthfully, like the famous ET finger, mine was pointing toward home, sending me a message to straighten up and pay attention to my body.

Perhaps it was the humor of the moment, the comfort level with my companion, my vulnerability. I was, after all sitting across from a first date, giving him the perpetual FINGER.

So I laid everything else on the table along with my unused chopsticks. I told him about my diet and celiac disease. And I confessed that I should not be eating at Chinese restaurants. I was a fraud, I admitted, teaching Chinese cooking when I shouldn't be eating the stuff.

I killed what was left of my glass of wine, imagining I had probably done the same to any chance for a second date. Not only was my finger damaged, my gut was a mess. I was weird inside and out, damaged goods.

To my surprise, two days later he invited me to his apartment for dinner. I hadn't scared off this doctor person. "I made you a gluten-free meal," he announced as he greeted me and my bandaged finger at the door.

I was blown away. Someone cared enough to cook a safe meal for *me*. The menu was chicken and rice and veggies. The pièce de

▶

▼

résistance was dessert, thumbprint cookies adapted from a recipe in the local newspaper. The moment I sank my teeth into those cookies, I knew I had a keeper! We were married in 1984 and have a son who is amazing and gifted and also has celiac disease. He often prefers to cook for his girlfriends rather than navigate a restaurant menu in the early days of dating. (The apple doesn't fall far from the tree!)

The cookie recipe resurfaced recently, and with it, many fond memories. Most of all, it reminded me of what it means to have good friends who go the extra mile to look out for one another. It's the kind of support that makes it easier to stay on a restrictive diet, the kind that makes a person feel special, not strange, protected, not peculiar.

Fitting in *is* a big deal. A lot of us worry more about what people think than about what's good for us. But after all these years, my advice to anyone whose friends don't take your diet seriously: "Get some new friends!" After all, real friends don't let friends eat gluten.

Dating

Dating and gluten-free can be a scary duo, scary enough so some people don't want to date at all. But you have to get out and enjoy yourself.

Here are a few ways to ease into the social scene. And don't limit yourself to dating. These tips will help you find your comfort zone with new friendships and social gatherings, too.

- Pick a place you are familiar with and where you feel safe ordering.
- Go out for a drink only so you get to know the person and feel comfortable before you have a meal together.
- Cook together. It's super romantic. Any girl loves a guy who can cook, and vice versa. It's a great activity and a wonderful way to get to know someone. Plus it's a healthier, easier way to manage the diet.
- Bring up the topic in a natural, not urgent way. These days, almost everyone knows someone who can't eat gluten.

- Go out with another celiac. See "Resources for the Twenty-Something" on page 266.
- Meet-up groups are a good way to meet others who need a gluten-free diet. You can take lessons from peers while you socialize.

Amie Valpone, a blogger friend at thehealthyapple.com, is in her early thirties and has more food allergies than a Chinese menu has dishes (including gluten, dairy, and most processed foods). She says it's easier to arrange to go to a museum, movie, or concert—nothing that involves food. She loves tea dates, too.

Pointers Your Date Needs to Know to Keep You Safe and Happy

- Don't keep smearing ChapStick or lip gloss on your lips and expect your date to pucker up. (Who knows what's in that gloss.)
- Never say, "Just try a little bit. It can't hurt you this one time." You won't get a second date.
- Never drink beer, then ask for a kiss.
- Be careful not to reach for the bread basket and let crumbs fall on your date's plate.
- Don't pick a restaurant without consulting your food-sensitive date. And *never* insist on pizza unless you know the restaurant serves gluten-free varieties, too.
- Don't butter your bread, then use the same knife to cut a piece of fish to share.
- Don't dip pita bread into the shared olive oil or hummus; or dip flour tortillas in shared salsa or guacamole.

Ways to Tell Whether Your Date Is a Keeper

- He or she rinses his or her mouth before kissing you.
- He or she asks you to pick the restaurant.
- You go to a house party together and he or she brings along gluten-free food.

- He or she cooks a meal or a treat that's safe for your diet.
- He or she brings you extra-large packages of Charmin for your birthday.

Resources for the Twenty-Something

Blogs and websites presented by and for the twenty-something abound. These bloggers offer a host of stories on gluten-free lifestyle, restaurant reviews, product information, and personal encounters. See Resources, page 311.

A Gluten Smooch: French (Bread) Kissing

Here's a question that seems as if it shouldn't need to be asked—but as with everything else to do with GFD, it's never that easy: Can I kiss my lover on the mouth? Well, of course, but do it carefully.

Just as you wouldn't lick the crumbs out of the bottom of a bread basket, nor should you explore your lover's mouth just after he or she has eaten a piece of crusty French bread or a beefy slice of pizza.

That's not to say you shouldn't get cozy with your companion if you want to. Just ask him or her to rinse or drink a bit of water before smooching.

And, hey, if you don't like your date all that much, French bread can be your savior. Pass the bread basket . . . then say you can't kiss someone who has just eaten gluten!

Let's Have THAT Talk

You might think this is the weirdest thing you've ever heard, but of course, kissing can be a source of cross-contamination. Crumbs on facial hair or entangled in a coiffed head of curls, gluten lingering on the lips and tongue—can all be potential quicksand for a gluten-sensitive or celiac person. (Maybe not so much for gluten avoiders.)

For the sake of your gut, give 'em the cheek when they go for the mouth. And it's okay to ask your date/partner to brush his or her teeth or wash up a bit before you get into some heavy-duty gluten smooching.

Sally's Story: Gluten-free Flowers

My friend Sally Ekus is also my literary agent. She has a sensitivity to several foods, including gluten, chicken eggs, cow dairy, and mustard. After many years of experiencing severe digestive issues, she finally began to narrow down the culprits when she was a freshman in college. Dating has always been a bit of an issue for Sally. "I hated explaining my diet, especially on a first date, which was often over a shared meal. It adds so much tension when you want to be casual and just get to know someone. Some topics really should be off limits yet I am forced to address them early on."

Today Sally is dating someone who looks after her diet even more than she does. He cooks for her and picks up foods he knows are "Sally-friendly." "He's a keeper," she says.

Her friend has completely changed how Sally feels about her allergies. He helps in the hunt for special food that's safe for her to eat. "It makes me feel special, and also really safe. I don't feel like an outcast, plus he chooses to order food to share with me."

"On one of our first dates he picked me up on the way to dinner and said, 'I hope it's okay. I want to try the tasting menu tonight.' I was immediately filled with anxiety as tasting menus are almost always off-limits for me. Before I could even respond, in his next breath he said that he had already called ahead and briefed the chef on my allergies. Not only was the chef creating a menu I could enjoy, but my date was going to have the same one as well. What a gift. For me, organizing a safe tasting menu is far better than sending flowers. I don't want flowers—I want love and safe food.

"When I am with him, my life is part of his. I don't have to substitute out something to make it work."

Whether you are involved with someone or speed dating, consider stocking up on disposable travel toothbrush kits and hand one to your date after eating and before you get romantic. If your date has a habit of smearing lip balm around the mouth, that, too, can be a source of gluten and another reason to kiss cautiously.

If this person is a keeper, you'll need to have a talk about these things as the relationship progresses. Think of it as gluten-free foreplay!

> My diet always comes up on a first date. It doesn't define me, but it's part of who I am. Once, I thought I had mentioned it because we went to a restaurant with a gluten-free menu. Obviously I hadn't. My date was eating gluten and I was eating gluten-free. Then he reached across with his fork to try my food. I slapped him away. We both had a good laugh after I explained why I was protecting my plate!
>
> —LINDSEY SCHNITT, A RECENT PENN STATE GRAD
> (SEE HER STORY, "WELL FED, WELL SCHOOLED," ON PAGE 250)

Body Balms, Gluten Smooching, and Lovemaking

Dr. Ruth might call kissing foreplay. I call it gluten smooching.

Wherever your tongue goes, the digestive tract follows. Gluten in skin care products is not generally a problem unless you have a wheat allergy and it extends to skin contact with wheat and gluten. Gluten absorbed through the skin goes into the bloodstream and not into the digestive system *unless* you lick it. Lipsticks and lip balms, facial creams, shampoos, conditioners, and skin lotions that come in contact with the mouth invite gluten in.

Without getting graphic, only you know which lotions you are using and what they are being used for. To get the most enjoyment out of your partner, avoid products that contain wheat, wheat germ oil, or oats.

By the time this is an issue, I hope you are familiar enough with your partner to go through his or her body products and make your diet a scintillating part of your relationship.

Can Gluten Affect Your Sex Life?

The answer is probably yes. First of all, you should not be eating gluten, and if you do, you might be feeling crappy, bloated, and tired. Excuse me, but who wants to get cozy while feeling bloated and crampy?

Aside from feeling yucky, we know a few specifics, too. Women with untreated celiac disease can suffer a wide array of reproductive issues (see "Infertility, Pregnancy, and Miscarriage," page 17).

A couple of small studies have looked at sexual satisfaction and celiac disease, too.

A small study in the *European Journal of Gastroenterology & Hepatology* indicates that if you are diagnosed with celiac disease and follow a gluten-free diet, it improves your sex drive. Maybe that's because you feel better, less tired, and more comfortable in your own skin.[1]

Another study found a similar link when it followed grown-up celiac children. In this one, researchers looked at three groups of young adults, all of whom had celiac disease. Some had followed the gluten-free diet since being diagnosed in childhood, some had adhered to a gluten-free diet for a year or more after diagnosis but then had reverted to a gluten-filled diet, and some had never followed the gluten-free diet.[2]

Those in the "never gluten-free" group had less interest in sex than did those in either of the other two groups. But those who followed the diet continually and those who had followed the diet for some of the time had a 5 to 7 percent higher interest in sex. So, if you have celiac disease or gluten sensitivity, stick to your gluten-free diet. It can improve your sex life.

If you are a gluten avoider, you may also find your energy level and interest in sex are related to abstaining from gluten.

A Roll in the Gluten-free Hay

Throughout this book we have discussed many things that the gluten-free lifestyle forces you to give up. Fortunately, sex is not one of them.

An active sex life may actually enhance your overall well-being by reducing stress, lowering your blood pressure, and releasing oxytocin and endorphins, which help reduce pain and discomfort, all while boosting your body's antibody response. It also burns calories, perhaps nature's antidote to too many gluten-free carbs.

Now that you've adopted a gluten-free diet, you are feeling energetic and attractive again, your hormones have normalized, your desires are rekindled, and you have those unexpected gaseous emissions under control. You have made it past the crumb and beer–cleaning timeout and have passed gluten-free first base. Now what? This is not that kind of a book, so the next step is up to you.

But here are some things you should know about sex the gluten-free way:

- Body fluids do not carry gluten.
- Allergic reactions may occasionally be associated with sexual activity, but are more likely reactions to other substances, such as latex, and in rare cases, semen.
- For your overall health, always take proper precautions to prevent STDs. And if products cause skin or mucosal irritation, (neither of which is due to gluten), seek alternative products.
- Lubricants, spermicidal/contraceptive jellies, condoms, foams, and sponges are generally gluten-free. As with cosmetics and other body lotions, unless you eat them, you will not have gluten issues. And if you are eating this stuff, what are you doing in the bedroom anyway?
- Edible underwear (Candypants and others) is made of either pressed candylike materials or candy pieces strung together. Who knew? If this option appeals to you, pick a brand with recognizable candies and check the labels. The same holds true for edible body oils and paints.
- For those who categorize body-applied foods as an essential food group, simple gluten-free choices include whipped cream, jam, and honey. But with the increase in bear attacks, honey may not be the best selection for camping trips.
- Although there is great variability from person to person, evidence suggests decreased fertility, decreased libido, and low energy levels in untreated individuals. So, you may think you cannot get pregnant. Don't be fooled. Now that your energy is increasing so is your chance of becoming pregnant. Check ingredients of oral contraceptive pills and other medications, if you choose them (see "Gluten and Medication," page 101).

Gut Reaction: Gluten-free Panties

The company I founded, Gluten Free Pantry, was an Internet pioneer. Our first website was launched in 1996. By 2003 we were pretty savvy at search engine optimization, a.k.a. getting to the top of the search engine listings. In the optimization process you repeatedly test the search engines to see how well your placement strategy is working. On one occasion we accidently entered "Gluten Free Panty." Well, even Google blushed and we got an eyeful of adult sites that pretty much ignored "gluten" and went right for the free panties. I often wondered whether I had gone into the wrong business.

Baby Love—More on Gluten Smooching

After courtship, comes marriage (maybe). And the next thing you know, there's an entire family with babies, children, and pets.

Who doesn't love kissing babies, especially your own? Nibbling those pudgy little hands, lips, ears, cheeks—it's all so delicious. And babies reciprocate. They stick their fingers in your mouth, grab your fingers, and share their food. Unless the baby is gluten-free, he or she has probably just devoured a handful of animal crackers, Cheerios, or teething biscuits. And now, you get to share.

Who thinks about this kind of stuff? But one day you kiss the baby on your way to work and by ten a.m., your tummy is hurting. Smooching even the older kids (think: Pop-Tarts and pancakes) can give you a hefty dose of gluten. Don't say no to gluten smooching. Just be sure to have them wipe the gluten off their hands and mouth before you kiss and hug.

The same goes for kissing your pet. Yes, some people kiss their animals on the mouth. (I'll admit I'm guilty, too.) Please wipe your pet's mouth after it's eaten and before you start smooching. This is really important if one of your kids is gluten-sensitive or celiac. Kids love to kiss their dogs on the lips (and dogs love to lick crumbs—gluten-free or not—from kids' faces). This hold true for cats and other critters, too.

Raising Your GF IQ:
The Birds and the Bees and the Gluten-free

How long do I need to wait to have sex after eating?

It's not like you need to wait for the pizza and French bread to fully digest. But do keep in mind that residual gluten can linger on the tongue, lips, and hands, and via crumbs in the hair and facial hair.

Rinsing the mouth, wiping the lips, washing the hands, and brushing hair and beards will help. If possible, ask your partner to brush his or her teeth, too.

Can my date catch what I have?

You might be mingling bodily fluids, but you can't intermingle genes. Gluten sensitivity, celiac disease, and wheat allergies are not contagious. The predisposition comes from within. It's not a virus or an infection. However, gluten-free food is so delicious, your date might want to have what you have—in a restaurant, that is.

What if I have a gluten attack while on a date?

There's nothing worse than getting sick on a date. But anyone could get a stomach bug or diarrhea and it's not even a gluten issue. Try not to take it too hard. This will pass. It's just a bummer to eat something on a date that makes you sick. Then you associate that person with your uncomfortable evening.

Excuse yourself and find a restroom—quickly. (I usually note the locations when I arrive, just in case.) If there's a lounge where you can rest for a few minutes, even better. Once you've regained your composure, tell your date you are not feeling well and you would like to go home. If you feel comfortable with that person, let him or her know you ate something that contained gluten.

If you really like this person, let him or her know how badly you feel about spoiling the evening and that you would like to cook dinner (or take the person out) to make up for it. This way you are also in control of the next get-together, diminishing the chances you'll get sick again.

When you've got to go: the big D and public restrooms.

If you are anything like me, you probably have a honing device in your brain that takes note of public restrooms wherever you go. (I also notice which ones seem the cleanest and largest. If I end up spending a long time in the bathroom, I don't want someone to keep knocking at the door, wondering when I'll be finished.)

If you need to go, grab an extra roll of toilet paper if you find one in the bathroom and line the toilet seat. Try to stay calm and take all the time you need. If you are with friends of the same sex, ask someone to bring you a bottle of water or a cup of tea. It sometimes helps.

What should I do when a server doesn't care about my diet?

You probably don't want to interrogate your server or challenge him or her in front of a casual date or casual friends. Quietly excuse yourself from the table and find the manager. Have a conversation about your diet, preferably in a spot that is not in view of your table. Say you need help and ask the manager to suggest things that might be safe. Let him or her know you've already spoken with a server whom you worry might not understand the severity of your diet. Point out your table and ask the manager to oversee your order and personally bring it to you. Worst-case, order a simple salad and a baked potato and enjoy the company.

What do I do when someone asks, "What happens when you eat gluten? Can I watch?"

They're joking, right? Do they really want to watch you barf all over and crap your pants? I don't think so. If your friends ask you this, get some new friends, honey. (For reinforcement, read "Friends Don't Let Friends Eat Gluten," page 261.)

14

Coping

What to Do When You're Gluten-ed

"Help! The other night I was at a dinner. They served cheese and crackers. They know I am gluten-intolerant. The hostess had gluten-free crackers for me, but she put them on the same plate with the wheat crisps. I thought they were all safe and did not think to ask until I consumed about four crackers. What would you do?" asked my friend Andrew.

I know exactly how he feels. Getting gluten-ed takes all the enjoyment out of socializing. Life's complacency evaporates and in its place, an uneasy, gnawing sensation sets in. You know something physically unpleasant is about to happen. It's as if a belt of dynamite was strapped to your waist and ready to go off at any moment.

Andrew thought about regurgitating, but ended up taking the hit the next day. He wondered whether there was another way to deal with the impending gluten reaction.

Unfortunately, there is no antidote or morning-after pill to ease the symptoms from ingesting gluten. Each person reacts differently and uses different techniques to ease the discomfort. Some people say they drink a lot of water. Some take digestive enzymes or lots of antacids. My twenty-something metropolitan son says he takes "a crap and a nap" and then feels better.

Despite all the improvements in the gluten-free marketplace, one thing hasn't changed. We have to take the hit when we accidentally eat gluten.

Relief When You Get Gluten-ed

Everyone's symptoms are different when gluten is accidentally ingested. However, many people's symptoms follow a predictable pattern . . . one that clues them in that they've eaten something with gluten. While nothing can prevent a reaction, you can try some of the remedies that may give you relief:

- Sleep it off.
- Take a walk. Light exercise helps.
- Drink lots of water.
- Take probiotics.
- Take GlutenEase (a digestive enzyme that does not prevent gut damage but may provide some relief of symptoms).
- Take a warm bath.
- Wear loose-fitting clothes if bloating is an issue.
- Take Tylenol (for a gluten headache).
- Avoid alcohol.
- Eat chicken soup or other warm soup.
- Drink ginger or mint tea.

Raising Your GF IQ:
Preventing a Glutening Meltdown

"My mother-in-law thinks I am just being fussy when I tell her I can't eat anything she makes," says a friend. "She thinks this gluten thing is all in my head. I feel so much better now that I have given up gluten, but this behavior gives me a new kind of pain. How do I handle her?"

Don't you wish you could strangle your MIL with a gluten-free pretzel? But it's important to keep the peace. The trick is to out-cook her. By that I mean, when you get together, take food that's safe and delicious. If you are up to the task, make a risotto, pasta dish, or casserole that is safe for your diet and enough to feed the whole group. Take a decadent dessert, too, one that you know will get rave reviews from everyone. At some point, your MIL will re-alize you take this diet seriously and she should as well. She will also notice that it's a manageable diet and delicious, too. Besides, she's probably a lousy cook who could benefit from a few pointers, gluten-free, of course.

I've been craving glazed doughnuts. It shouldn't hurt once in a while, right?

No! Don't fall on your sword for gluten, my friend. Whether you are gluten-sensitive or have celiac disease, (gluten avoiders, too, should take note), please let your good senses prevail. You'll pay the price later if you eat that doughnut now. Have something decadent that's also safe. Hot fudge sundae, anyone?

By the way, you don't need to cheat to eat some pretty good doughnuts. The recipe is on page 181.

What do I do when people say, "Just this once can't hurt?"

Don't let the downers wear you down by waving a forkful of decadent chocolate cake in your face. Don't you wonder what they have to gain by offering this stellar advice? Do they want you to share the calories so they won't feel guilty? Do they think the gluten thing is all in your head? Take the serious approach and say, "No, thank you. Even a bite would make me very sick." Or take the approach I might use and bite (maybe just push) the hand that's trying to feed you as you growl, "That little bite will make me crap my pants."

No Gluten, No Tootin'—The Gas Thing

First the disclaimer. I can't promise that you won't have any gas once you give up gluten. But the title is one of those penned by the Scotch and Taco bunch that helped name this book (if you've forgotten this list—intentionally or otherwise, revisit it on page xxvi). Everyone has gas. It's natural. But sometimes, when you have celiac disease or gluten sensitivity, it feels as if your whole life revolves around a bloated belly and unpredictable gaseous emissions. That's not natural. This section is about helping you to manage the gas and those embarrassing moments. Granted, this is a really delicate subject. But it's just you and me here and your secret is safe.

I think those of us with celiac disease and gluten sensitivity experience gas in stereo. Our digestive system may empty more slowly, allowing for more bloating . . . and the crescendo is the ear-splitting gaseous emissions as the digestive process proceeds. That's especially true if we've eaten something we should not eat.

I've lost count of the number of times the word *bloating* is mentioned in this book. It can be a symptom of celiac disease and gluten sensitivity and DH. What do you suppose causes that feeling? If you guessed, gas, you are right. *Flatulence, farts, passing wind, passing gas.* These are all terms that we have committed to memory but are afraid to talk about. It's the embarrassing stuff that makes people with celiac disease lose their sense of humor.

Gut Gas?

In the comfort and safety of these pages, I say, "Let 'er rip." But you can't do that in public, or at least you try not to. Sometimes the discomfort is overwhelming. It can ruin a date or an evening out. You might find the need to excuse yourself and go outside, to your car, or to a bathroom for a while to try to relieve some of the pressure.

Yes, "embarrassing" and "uncomfortable" come to mind.

Cut Back or Cut Loose: A Few Ways to Reduce Gas and Bloating.

- **Avoid gluten** (the obvious).
- **Take a digestive enzyme.** GlutenEase is an over-the-counter product that helps diminish symptoms if you accidentally eat gluten. (It does not prevent an autoimmune response, if you are celiac.)
- **Take CVS Pharmacy Beanaid Enzyme Supplement**, an OTC supplement that helps to relieve bloating and indigestion from eating beans, broccoli, and seeds. Bean-zyme is a similar product that touts the same benefits and ingredients. (Beano is not safe for a gluten-free diet.)
- **Take a daily probiotic.** Probiotics are friendly bacteria of which we don't make sufficient amounts on our own (for more on probiotics, see page 71).

- **Avoid dairy products or cut back on them.** As many as 50 percent of people with celiac disease and many with gluten sensitivity also have a sensitivity to dairy. The amount of dairy tolerated depends on the individual. Take Lactaid pills when you eat dairy to help break down the lactose or avoid all dairy products. (Not all Lactaid products are gluten-free, so check with the manufacturer.)
- **Avoid or reduce the amount of high-fiber foods,** such as broccoli, Brussels sprouts, cauliflower, legumes, and such fruits as apples and prunes.
- **Avoid carbonated beverages and chewing gum.** Both add extra air to your digestive system and that has to come out someplace.
- **Avoid artificial sweeteners.** While artificial sweeteners are mostly gluten-free, such products as xylitol and sorbitol have been shown to double normal gas production by fueling the growth of bacteria in the large intestine. This is a double whammy if you chew gum that is artificially sweetened.
- **Try simethicone products.** Over-the-counter products, such as Gas-X, help break up the bubbles in gas. These offer some relief, but results are inconclusive. Check labels first as not all of these medications are gluten-free.
- **Use activated charcoal tablets.** Take them before and after a meal. They're available in natural food stores and many drugstores. Check labels first, as not all products are gluten-free.
- **Drink a lot of water.** It helps reduce the bubbles of air and moves the food through your system more quickly.
- **Drink peppermint tea.** Peppermint is a great, natural digestive aid. Avoid it, however, if you have acid reflux, as it can exacerbate those symptoms.
- **Take a walk.** After eating, a little light exercise helps get things moving.

Note: About GlutenEase and other digestive enzymes. Don't be one of those folks who says, "I can have a little gluten. I'll just take a digestive enzyme and be fine." Although these can mask symptoms, they are not a free pass to eat gluten. You'll still be doing harm, especially if you have celiac disease or one of the other related autoimmune disorders.

Disaster Plan, Take 2

Disaster preparedness sounds like an oxymoron, but in this day of Global Weirdness, natural disaster can strike anytime, anywhere. Hurricane, tornado, flood, blizzard, earthquake, or fire, you name it. And it's disaster-times-two for someone on a gluten-free diet, unless he or she has a supply of safe food on hand.

Picture this. You're safe and sound in your own house one minute, and the next, there's a flood and it's filling the basement and tickling the top of the stairs that lead to the first floor. The toilets don't flush, the electricity is off, and the phone is about to die. All of a sudden, home doesn't look so comforting anymore. A police boat comes by and someone tells you to evacuate to higher ground. The announcer says gather some belongings and your medications and he'll be back to pick you up in five minutes. He'll take you to a shelter where you will have food, water, and a place to sleep. He doesn't mention that safe gluten-free food is a pipe dream and that you will need to stand in line to use a toilet.

In the blink of an eye, this scenario can be yours, your salvation and your worst nightmare rolled into one.

If you are anything like me, you've been lulled into thinking, "This can't happen to me."

But over an eighteen-month period, five weather-related disasters hit in my own backyard in nothing-ever-happens-here Connecticut.

I hope this message resonates with you. There's nothing worse than being overtaken by a gluten attack in a shelter where water and Porta Potties are rationed.

Be Proactive. Have a Plan.

Let's put together an emergency kit and some tips to help you stay safe and comfortable, whether you are stranded at home or need to grab-and-go to a shelter.

Avoiding Bread Lines

Here's the good news about preparing for a disaster. When a hurricane or blizzard is brewing, you probably won't be one of those waiting in line at the grocery store to stock up on bread and mac and cheese. Instead of fighting over the last loaf, you will be stocked up ahead.

The Red Cross recommends a seventy-two-hour (three-day) supply of food and water, but with all the extreme weather we've been having lately, I suggest you have a five-day supply of safe food at the ready.

Reality Check

The Red Cross and other emergency groups are fully stocked with peanut butter nabs, juice, water, and sandwiches, but they have very little available for people on special diets. In fact, FEMA recommends keeping a portable bag or box near a door and filling it with a supply of safe foods that you can grab quickly if you are evacuated.

Sheltering at Home

Handy Equipment—a Generator

If you are in an area where the electricity goes out for an extended period of time, consider investing in a generator. They come in all sizes, prices, and capacities. To me, the most important reason to have a generator is to keep a refrigerator going. A working refrigerator means gluten-free breads, meats, and other perishable foods can be stored safely for an extended period. And having a good supply of food affords a sense of comfort when everything else seems out of control.

A generator can keep the heat and hot water going, too. If you are a hearty soul who is accustomed to "roughing it," you might not see the need for these features. Personally, I like my basic comforts.

Cooking Alternatives

There's a lot to be said for having a camping stove or grill. These can be a lifesaver and can mean the difference between a hot cup of coffee and a cold can of soup. If you have either a grill or a stove and a cast-iron skillet, you have a well-equipped survival kitchen. You can make a batch of pancakes for breakfast, warm cans of soup for lunch, even grill sandwiches and eggs, or heat up a dehydrated meal for dinner.

Can Opener

Under "Stocking Your Gluten-Free Pantry" we'll talk about stockpiling cans of soup, beans, even chicken, stews, chili, and SPAM. It's great if these packages are equipped with flip-top lids, but not all companies manufacture that way. A basic can opener can make dinner happen. In fact, tuck away two lightweight ones so there's no cross-contamination.

Paper Plates, Cups, and Plastic Utensils

You can eat out of the can but it might be difficult to have milk and cereal that way. A supply of paper and plastic products can bring a level of comfort to home.

Food Supplies

An ice chest or operating refrigerator means you can keep a supply of milk, meat, and gluten-free bread on hand. (Keep a couple of loaves of prepared bread in the freezer. Even if the power goes out, these will thaw and keep for several days. Just remember to eat this bread first.) When supplies run out, you'll want to dig into your stash of crackers, dehydrated or canned meats, and powdered milk or protein.

Your stay-at-home pantry can include cans of beans, soups, and jars of peanut butter. Note that these will not work well in a portable emergency kit, as they can weigh you down. (See "Camping Foods That Do Double Duty" on page 315.)

On-the-Run-Evacuation Plans

You won't be able to bring much of the aforementioned equipment and supplies with you if you are evacuated. Put together a grab-and-go box of safe, lightweight gluten-free foods for this purpose.

Make your box as self-sufficient as possible. Going to a shelter is like communal camping in a tent for fifty-plus. It's likely you will not be catered to. You could have access to boiling water for dehydrated foods but still have to wait for a bowl or spoon. Bring them with you.

Think Outside the Box

Instead of storing supplies in cardboard boxes (think: soggy and mildewed), many folks pack survival items in old backpacks and hang them on hooks by the door and in a place where they are likely to stay dry in case of a flood and are easy to grab as you leave the house. Some people even keep a survival pack or box in the trunk of the car. However, you may not be able to travel by car, so make sure the box or backpacks are light enough to carry.

Outfit your box with:

- An inexpensive can opener or two
- A few paper or plastic bowls and some plastic spoons
- A roll of toilet paper
- Enough medication for several days, plus a copy of prescriptions
- **Gluten-free bread.** Many brands do not travel well. Pick shelf-stable, vacuum-sealed breads with an extended shelf life (visit Dr. Schär, schar.com, and Ener-G foods, ener-g.com).
- **Crackers.** These are light to carry, well packaged, and a great alternative to breads. Many companies make gluten-free crackers, including Crunchmaster, Glutino, Mary's Gone Crackers, and Dr. Schär. And crackers have a much longer shelf life than breads (up to a year).
- **Pancake mixes.** A great source of chew factor. As a mix, these keep for a long time and, in a pinch, can be made with water and without eggs. Use them as wraps, too. You can even make pancakes over a campfire or grill, too. Glutino Instant Pancake Mix, a powdered mix in a lightweight container, is ideal. Just add water when you want pancakes.

Lightweight Foods

Asian rice noodles

Bouillon (Herb-Ox) great for flavoring rice, rice noodles, and other foods

Cereals (bulky but lightweight)

Dried soups

Dried coconut

Dried fruits and nuts

Freeze-dried vegetables and fruits

Gluten-free pasta

Gluten-free pretzels

Instant coffee

Instant gluten-free oatmeal

Kale chips

Meats and other protein sources (e.g., Shelton turkey jerky)

Peanut or other nut butter, preferably in squeezable pouches

Powdered milk and cream

Protein powder

Snack bars

Tea bags

Tuna and salmon in shelf-stable pouches

I mentioned this earlier, but it bears repeating here: Several companies specialize in camping and on-the-go shelf-stable gluten-free foods. They are perfect for survival kits, too. Go to "Camping," page 217, for the list.

Shelf Life Matters

Be sure to rotate your supplies. Pick the shortest shelf life as a gauge and throw a Thank-Goodness-We-Didn't-Need-This Party to use up foods before they spoil. Before you chow down, make a list so you'll know what needs to be replaced.

Quick Meal Ideas

Mix protein powder into cups of applesauce.

Reconstitute Asian rice noodles with bouillon and dehydrated veggies and meat for a hearty meal.

Mix dried fruit into instant oatmeal for a nutrition boost.

Emergency Kits Reminders

Store your emergency grab-and-go kit up HIGH.

Pack lightly. When making the list for your disaster kit, consider whether a dehydrated or shelf-stable pouch versions of each product is available. Think: powdered milk versus shelf-stable cartons; dehydrated meats instead of canned versions; dried fruits and fruit rollups versus canned or fresh fruit.

Start building your box or backpack with freeze-dried and dehydrated products, products geared to emergency preparedness. Once in place, fill in with canned foods only when the dehydrated versions are not available.

Avoid packing family-size portions. Although they might seem less expensive and more practical, the packaging might be cumbersome and it may be difficult to store leftovers, cooked or uncooked. Don't waste valuable real estate on family-size packaging.

You might not have access to transportation, so make sure the kit is small enough and light enough to carry it a good distance. A knapsack or light rolling duffle works well.

Pack utensils. Put plastic utensils, a paring knife, and a can opener in a resealable plastic bag. Include a box of disinfectant wipes or hand sanitizer and a small bag of first-aid supplies.

Water proof. Assume that everything might get wet during an emergency. Wrap food that could become damaged by water in waterproof bags. These bags can double as trash and storage bags once you are settled in your shelter.

Don't forget vitamins and medications. It is essential that these be in waterproof packaging.

Label products that are safe for people with allergies and keep track of the packaging. This is especially true if you have single-serve items in one larger package. If foods are separated from the original package, you still know they are safe.

Cross-Contamination and Survival

Without running water to wash utensils, pots, and plates, it's nearly impossible to cut out all cross-contamination. Sani-wipes can clean hands but utensils cannot be cleaned as thoroughly. Consider making everything gluten-free or segregating out certain knives, boards, or pans for gluten-filled foods and keeping them separate.

Gluten-free Food Emergency Suppliers

Some naturally gluten-free foods are available through the Red Cross and the Salvation Army.

Three efforts are under way within the gluten-free community, to help supply emergency foods.

- GlutenFreeDee.com is run by Dee Valdez in Loveland, Colorado, and is national in scope.
- Pierce's Pantry, piercespantry.com, supplies food banks in Massachusetts and is partnering the Celiac Support Association (CSA) to take its endeavors to a national level.
- CSA runs a natural disaster emergency gluten-free hotline: 1-888-272-4255.

Label systems for products are available through Kemnitz Family Kitchen Gluten-free Labels, kfk-enjoy.com, and kidcals.com.

Pain in the Pocketbook

So, you think you had pain before you went on a gluten-free diet? You might feel better, but now your pocketbook may begin to hurt when you start buying gluten-free products. This diet is expensive. Never mind sticker shock, this is gluten shock.

"There are a few contributing factors to the premium price of gluten-free food versus their gluten-filled counterparts. First, many of the ingredients that are used to replace gluten-full ingredients can be more expensive. Gluten-full flours are generally more commodity priced, whereas a specialty gluten-free replacement ingredient is more premium priced. This can be based on availability of that unique ingredient or based on processing and storage methods to reduce the risk of cross-contamination or based on the documentation that we require to ensure the ingredient is gluten-free. Additionally, brands like Glutino invest a significant amount of money in testing to ensure our products are gluten-free. Glutino has a test-and-hold policy, meaning that no product ships until we receive third-party test results that the product is gluten-free."

—LAURA KUYKENDALL, DIRECTOR OF MARKETING, GLUTINO

Raising Your GF IQ:
Why Is Gluten-free Food So Expensive?

- The cost of a loaf of bread can be double or triple the price of regular bread. The from-scratch ingredients have to be sourced from manufacturers that can verify their products are safe, too.
- Gluten-free pasta is very expensive. Very few brands are made in the United States. On top of expensive ingredients, you pay the cost of importing it, too. Several fresh artisan brands are made in this country. These are delicious but you'll pay dearly.
- Manufacturing facilities are small. Even with all the demand for gluten-free products, we're not talking mega mass production here.
- Delivering fresh-tasting products to the consumer is challenging. Gluten-free foods tend to spoil (no preservatives) or dry out (no gluten) as they are shipped across the country.
- Products are fragile and crush easily. Packaging can be difficult and costly.
- Gluten-free companies often test each batch of products before releasing it to consumers. More ca-ching.

Have I Got a Deal for You: Ways to Save

Gluten-free has become big business with plenty of competition. Deals and coupons abound. That's great news for people on a GFD.

Since we don't have a choice, we might as well get the best deal we can on this diet.

Here are a few ways to save:

- Stock up when items go on sale or when you have a coupon.
- Get coupons and promotions. Sign up on Facebook pages or websites of your favorite products. See Resources, page 316, for other money-saving websites.
- Buy in bulk. Amazon.com and BobsRedMill.com offer great savings when you buy in bulk.
- If you are a baker, buy cases or 5-pound bags of the flours.
- Amazon.com sells Bob's Red Mill products, other brands of flours, and hundreds of other gluten-free items. Shipping is usually free if you join its Amazon Prime members group.
- Bob's Red Mill offers promotions online, but shipping can be hefty.
- Odd Job Lot, Ocean State Job Lot, Walmart, and Price Chopper stock an abundance of gluten-free food at good prices.
- Explore Indian markets. Traditional gram flour is made from chickpeas and is safe (note: this is not graham flour, which contains wheat). Juar flour is jowar or sorghum flour; urid flour is lentil flour.
- Investigate Asian markets: Glutinous rice flour is finely ground sweet rice. No gluten here. Chickpea flour and rice flour are also available at good prices. Although there are no guarantees that these are free from cross-contamination, very little wheat is processed in Asia.
- Asian markets can be a great source of rice noodles and buckwheat soba noodles. *But don't take a chance if the label is not written in English. Some of these noodles also contain wheat flour.*

Some Cautionary Notes

- Buying flours at ethnic markets can be a source of irresistible bargains and risky business, too, unless you can read the labels. Be a savvy shopper.
- Supermarkets and natural food stores often sell flours and grains in bulk grocery bins. But don't be tempted to purchase your flours this way. Scoops may be shared and bins can become cross-contaminated.

More Cost-Cutting Ideas

Buy Naturally Gluten-free

Fresh vegetables, fruits, fish, dairy, and meats are naturally gluten-free—and healthy, to boot. These don't increase your budget, as you would be buying them anyway. Seems like the best of all worlds, doesn't it?

From Scratch

Instead of buying commercial mixes or prepared foods, make your own. Make your own flour blends and mixes in large batches and store them in bins so they are ready for all your baking needs. (See more about flours and blends on page 164.)

Deep Freeze

Store individual-size portions of baked goods in the freezer until you need them. This is perfect for busy families, especially those where the gluten-free person is a child. Freeze soups, sauces, and some entrées, too.

Second That

Many people on a gluten-free diet buy a second refrigerator or freezer to store all their flours, blends, and baked goods. Make sure to catalog items and date and label them so your gluten-free treasures don't get lost in a frozen abyss.

When the Gluten-free Diet Breaks the Bank

Gluten-free food can truly break the bank if you are on a limited income. But help is available. Check your local food pantry or the regional food bank. Let the staff know you will need gluten-free food on a regular basis and go over a list of products you will need.

Two gluten-free organizations have been working with local food banks to supply gluten-free food.

- GlutenFreeDee.com is run by Dee Valdez in Loveland, Colorado, who works with twenty or more food pantries across the United States.

- Pierce's Pantry, piercespantry.com, supplies ten food banks in Massachusetts. Twenty-something Pierce Keegan has partnered with the Celiac Support Association (CSA) to take his endeavors to a national level.

Take It Off Your Taxes

If you have a diagnosis of celiac disease, you can deduct the difference between gluten-free food and gluten-filled food when you do your income taxes (under medical deductions). But it means keeping good records and recording every purchase. And you'll need medical documentation, too, especially if you are audited.

You can also deduct the cost of transportation to buy the product or shipping if it comes by mail order. However, to take the deduction, beginning January 1, 2013, the total of all your medical expenses has to be more than 10 percent of your adjusted gross income. Talk to a tax accountant to determine whether you qualify.

Gluten-sensitive people have a few more hoops to jump through to get a tax break. Because this is a relatively new condition, you may have arrived at the diet by default, not by diagnosis, and documentation might be scarce. You'll need to find a health practitioner who can establish your need for a GFD. A letter from a naturopathic physician can be a good choice if conventional medicine is not. But check with the IRS to make sure it will accept this diagnosis before you start saving records.

Gluten avoiders, I'm afraid you are out of luck when it comes to taking this diet off your taxes. You'll have to look for other deductions—business lunch, anyone?

Special Circumstances:
Hospital Stays, Retirement Communities,
Rehab Facilities, and Nursing Homes

Institutional food service can seem terrifying for someone on a GFD. So many layers of employees. So many shifts. And so many other issues to worry about. But you need to make the effort and ask a relative to help you ensure that you can eat safely during your stay. Maintaining your GFD is part of your overall health and healing.

The good news is that an increasing number of institutions are aware of the GFD and some have even gone through a training program offered by NFCA or GIG (see Resources, page 306). Happily, many major food service suppliers now carry gluten-free food items. They are readily available to institutional kitchens. Nonetheless, some institutions are terrified to incorporate a gluten-free diet in their food plan. If they do, it's basic, plain, flavorless food. Be persistent.

Try to meet with the head of food service and the dietitian before you go into the hospital or move to a retirement community or a nursing home. Select safe food options and establish a diet plan. Get a printout of the menu you will be receiving so you can cross-check when your food is served. Switches happen.

Depending on the length of your stay, review this plan in one or two weeks to make sure everyone is still in agreement and the gluten-free person is happy. (Hopefully, if this is a hospital stay, you are home by now!)

Provide labels for your food and post signs in your room or at your bed as reminders.

If this is a nursing home stay, loved ones should emphasize the importance of the GFD to staff. Having gluten-free food can help decrease or alleviate confusion and dementia and improve bowel control and overall comfort all of which can change the outcome for a nursing home patient and caregivers (see "Suddenly Celiac: Seniors and Celiac Disease," page 24).

Military Service:
A GI Matter of a Different Kind

Hats off to the folks who serve in the military. But if you need a GFD, this might not be the life for you.

First of all, military service and celiac disease are mutually exclusive. The Department of Defense "Directive on Physical Standards for Appointment, Enlistment, or Induction," DODD 6130.3, specifically mentions celiac sprue as one of the conditions that exclude a person from serving.

It makes sense. The military does not procure or handle gluten-free food. That might not be a problem in the United States, where you can keep a stash of safe food at the ready and supplement with eggs and baked potatoes from the mess hall. But imagine being deployed to a place where you don't have those options and rely on MREs (Meals Ready to Eat) from a mess tent. Most are not gluten-free and being seriously celiac could jeopardize good health and the safety of those around. Imagine your having to be in the latrine while your unit is fighting or engaged in field exercises. As with everything, there are waivers, especially if you have a skill that the military needs, were diagnosed after joining the military service, and if you have a desk job in a location where you can buy gluten-free food.

The situation comes up from time to time when a military person is diagnosed with celiac disease after beginning his or her military career. It certainly limits the options for assignments and might be a reason for separation from the service (your choice or theirs).

For one person's experience with the GFD and military life, read *Gluten Free in Afghanistan*, a memoir by Captain B. Donald Andrasik, who enlisted in the Maryland National Guard and was deployed to Kandahar, Afghanistan, for a year.

If you are gluten-sensitive or gluten-free by choice, you'll need to weigh the pros and cons of choosing this lifestyle. Although your reasons for being gluten-free are not specifically spelled out in the DOD regulations, you'll face the same challenges in maintaining your diet and your health.

If you are looking for ways to serve your country, there are other options. How about the US Public Health Service?

15

Living Well

Final Thoughts on a Gluten-free Life Well Lived

As you've noticed, gluten-free is much more than a diet. It has a beginning (the diagnosis), but no end. This regimen creeps into every other aspect of life and travels with you to its outer edges. An exotic safari may be that much better because the cook made you gluten-free bread over the camp stove. A bond of friendship might be stronger for the gluten molecule that is absent and the gluten-free treats brought to you instead. A family wedding might be that much more meaningful because the bride and groom thought to include gluten-free options for their guests.

Although this book goes into those places and more, it's really just a beginning or, as the celiac docs like to say, "the tip of the celiac iceberg." I hope it provides you with fodder to begin or add to your journey to live well the gluten-free way.

As you start cooking, monitor your health, and maintain close tabs on your diet or your child's diet, you're going to continue to do your own research. As you do, here are just a few things to keep in mind.

Raising Your GF IQ:
Finding Information on the Internet

These days we all do most of our research on the Internet. It's a great resource for everything related to diagnosis, diet, and even survival.

But the information highway is only as good as its drivers. When an "expert" tells you something that doesn't ring true, it's a good thing to double-check your references.

See whether the same information appears on sites you trust. Rely first on medical sites (the celiac medical centers, PubMed, and NIH, for instance). Check patient support group sites for lifestyle issues. If a medical article is quoted, read the abstract (at pubmed.com).

Check the writer's credentials as well as the site. If the person has a degree in home economics and is recommending vitamins, move on.

Check the dates. Some information is very old but still gets repeated on blogs throughout cyberspace. Use the latest sources for your resources.

Here's one example of how a cyber myth gets passed around. This one relates to a rumor that coffee was "cross-reactive" for people with gluten issues. I love coffee so this really stirred me up. The same statement was repeated on several blogs. I discovered these bloggers had all attended a conference in which the lecturer warned of that connection. A few more clicks and I discovered the lecturer had a web page. I checked his credentials. He called himself "doctor." Did he have a PhD in food chemistry or was he an MD? Hidden in his web page was a reference to "DC" which I had to look up elsewhere. It turns out he is a doctor of chiropractic. In the comments, I noticed that people who had credentials that he was missing, said there was no truth to his statement. Coffee is fine for a GFD. See how easily we can be sidetracked on the Internet?

Note: Be wary of sites that claim to "cure" your gluten issues with a pill or a proprietary treatment, too. They do exist. I hope I've instilled you with enough gluten sensibility to help you separate good information from shaky claims.

Beth's Basic Rules for
Living Well the Gluten-free Way

I try not to impose a lot of rules on myself. Nothing is cut and dried in a land where every breath is framed by a special diet. But here are a few that I can impart—words of encouragement, really—as you venture down this gluten-free highway:

1. Learn everything you can about your diagnosis and the diet.
2. Don't ever assume you've learned it all. There's always more, and products and preparations *will* change.
3. Read ingredient labels carefully and double-check with manufacturers if you have concerns. (See Rule #2.)
4. Don't assume. Ask detailed questions about food preparation when in another home or restaurant.
5. Don't be shy. Find ways to bring up the conversation, whether it's with a host, a date, a friend, or a server in a restaurant. (We can work on that last one together. See "Restaurant Dining with Training Wheels," page 207.)
6. Forgive others who make mistakes when preparing something for you to eat. It's truly not the first thing on everyone's mind.
7. Use every experience as an opportunity to educate someone.
8. Embrace this mantra: *Just in case.* Carry something with you *just in case* there's nothing to eat where you are going.
9. Have a backup plan. Just as you need an emergency plan in case of fire or bad weather, have options for safe food, too.
10. Be upbeat. No whining or bitching, please.
11. Passive-aggressive behavior goes both ways, just like the swinging doors in a restaurant. And the server has the upper hand. He or she gets to decide what goes on your plate.
12. Be grateful and appreciative. Thank people who have gone out of their way to help you with your diet even if the choice was not ultimately safe or to your liking. (See Rule #10.)
13. Embrace comic relief: A good sense of humor makes this a lifestyle that you can embrace, rather than a life sentence. In case your

smile is missing, these websites are guaranteed to help you find it again:

Glutendude.com

Glutenfreeoptimist.com

Glutenismybitch.com

Michael Bihovsky's "One Grain More" (on YouTube)

14. If nothing else, remember this: You are truly the master of your universe when it comes to the GFD. You decide if you want to be the victor or the victim. It's up to you.

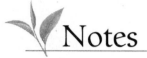# Notes

CHAPTER 1. ESSENTIAL THINGS YOU NEED TO KNOW ABOUT CELIAC DISEASE

1. Alessio Fasano, MD, et al., "Prevalence of Celiac Disease in At-Risk and Not-At-Risk Groups in the United States: A Large Multicenter Study," *Archives of Internal Medicine* 163, no. 3 (February 2003): 286–92.

2. A. Rubio-Tapia et al., "The Prevalence of Celiac Disease in the United States," *American Journal of Gastroenterology* 107, no. 10 (October 2012): 1538–44.

3. University of Chicago Center for Celiac Disease website, www.cureceliac .org.

4. Peter H. R. Green, MD, and Rory Jones, *Celiac Disease: A Hidden Epidemic*, Revised and Updated Edition, copyright © 2006, 2010 by Peter H. R. Green, MD, and Rory Jones, 116. Courtesy of HarperCollins Publishers.

5. F. Dickerson et al., "Markers of Gluten Sensitivity and Celiac Disease in Recent-Onset Psychosis and Multi-Episode Schizophrenia," *Biological Psychiatry*, May 14, 2010.

6. N. G. Cascella et al., "Increased Prevalence of Transglutaminase 6 Antibodies in Sera from Schizophrenia Patients," *Schizophrenia Bulletin*, July 2013.

7. Tetsuhide Ito, MD, PhD, and Robert T. Jensen, MD, "Association of Long-term Proton Pump Inhibitor Therapy with Bone Fractures and Effects on Absorption of Calcium, Vitamin B_{12}, Iron, and Magnesium," *Current Gastroenterology Reports* 12, no. 6 (December 2010): 448–57.

8. U. Peters et al., "Causes of Death in Patients with Celiac Disease in a Population-Based Swedish Cohort," *Archive of Internal Medicine* 163, no. 13 (July 14, 2003): 1566–72.

9. D. Martinelli et al., "Reproductive Life Disorders in Italian Celiac Women: A Case-Control Study," BMC *Gastroenterology*, August 6, 2010.

10. Hugh James Freeman, "Adult Celiac Disease in the Elderly," *World Journal of Gastroenterology* 14, no. 45 (December 7, 2008): 6911–14.

11. Shadi Rashtak, MD, and Joseph A. Murray, MD, "Celiac Disease in the Elderly," *Gastroenterology Clinics of North America* 38, no. 3 (September 2009): 433–46.

12. Y. Lurie et al., "Celiac Disease Diagnosed in the Elderly," Journal of Clinical Gastroenterology 42, no. 1 (January 2008): 59–61.

CHAPTER 2.
GETTING TESTED FOR CELIAC DISEASE

1. Arnold Han et al., "Dietary Gluten Triggers Concomitant Activation of CD4+ and CD8+ αβ T Cells and γδ T Cells in Celiac Disease," *Proceedings of the National Academy of Sciences of the U.S.*, June 26, 2013, www.pnas.org.

2. A. Rubio-Tapia et al., "ACG Clinical Guidelines: Diagnosis and Management of Celiac Disease," *American Journal of Gastroenterology*, May 2013.

3. Anneli Ivarsson et al., "Prevalence of Childhood Celiac Disease and Changes in Infant Feeding," *Pediatrics*, February 18, 2013, 10.1542/peds.2012-1015.

4. "Breastfeeding and the Use of Human Milk," policy statement from the American Academy of Pediatrics Policy 115, no. 2:496.

5. Peter H. R. Green, MD, and Rory Jones, *Celiac Disease: A Hidden Epidemic*, Revised and Updated Edition, copyright © 2006, 2010 by Peter H. R. Green, MD, and Rory Jones, 179. Courtesy of HarperCollins Publishers.

CHAPTER 3.
A BROADER SPECTRUM
OF GLUTEN-RELATED DISORDERS

1. Anna Sapone et al., "Spectrum of Gluten-Related Disorders: Consensus on New Nomenclature and Classification," *BMCMedicine*, February 7, 2012, www.biomedcentral.com.

2. Ibid.

3. Ibid.

4. N. M. Lau et al., "Markers of Celiac Disease and Gluten Sensitivity in Children with Autism," PLOS-One, June 18, 2013, plosone.org, 8(6):e66155.

5. T. A. Kabbani et al., "Patients with Celiac Disease Have a Lower Prevalence of Non-Insulin-Dependent Diabetes Mellitus and Metabolic Syndrome," *Gastroenterology*, May 2013.

CHAPTER 5.
THE DIET'S THE MEDICINE (FOR NOW)

1. Moises Velasquez-Manoff, "Who Has the Guts for Gluten?," *New York Times*, February 23, 2013.

2. Christine Boyd, "Love Your Gut: The Startling Role of Intestinal Flora in Food Allergy and Celiac Disease," *Living Without* magazine, Aug/Sept 2013; Michael Pollan, "Some of My Best Friends Are Germs," *New York Times* magazine, May 15, 2013.

CHAPTER 6. GLUTEN 101

1. Van Waffle, "Bob Anderson: Searching for a Cure for Celiac Disease," *Gluten-free Living* magazine, May/June 2013, 50.

2. Carlo Catassi et al., "A Prospective, Double-Blind, Placebo-Controlled Trial to Establish a Safe Gluten Threshold for Patients with Celiac Disease," *American Journal of Clinical Nutrition* 85 (2007): 160–66.

3. Justin R. Hollon et al., "Trace Gluten Contamination May Play a Role in Mucosal and Clinical Recovery in a Subgroup of Diet-Adherent Non-Responsive Celiac Disease Patients," BMC *Gastroenterology*, February 28, 2013, 13:40 doi:10.1186/1471-230X-13-40, www.biomedcentral.org.

CHAPTER 7.
GLUTEN, GLUTEN EVERYWHERE!

1. "Omission Beer Offers Additional Details About Proprietary Brewing Process," www.businesswire.com.

2. Michelle L. Colgrave, Hareshwar Goswami, Crispin A. Howitt, and Gregory J. Tanner, "What Is in a Beer? Proteomic Characterization and Relative Quantification of Hordein (Gluten) in Beer," *Journal of Proteome Research*, October 17, 2011.

3. Ibid.

4. Brent Hunsberger, "Gluten-Removed or Gluten-free, Craft Brew Alliance Presses Omission Beer's Case," *Oregonian*, June 8, 2013.

5. Ibid.

6. Interim Policy on Gluten Content Statements in the Labeling and Advertising of Wines, Distilled Spirits, and Malt Beverages, May 24, 2012, www.ttb.gov.

7. Catassi et al., "A Prospective, Double-Blind, Placebo-Controlled Trial," 160–66.

8. "Gluten in Cosmetics: What You Need to Know," bettermedicine.com, January 17, 2013.

CHAPTER 8. FOOD SHOPPING

1. Sabrina Tavernise, "F.D.A. Sets a Standard on Labeling 'Gluten Free'," *New York Times*, August 2, 2013.

2. Peter H. R. Green, MD, and Rory Jones, *Celiac Disease: A Hidden Epidemic*, Revised and Updated Edition, copyright © 2006, 2010 by Peter H. R. Green, MD, and Rory Jones, 46. Courtesy of HarperCollins Publishers.

CHAPTER 11. GETTING OUT: WHAT YOU NEED TO KNOW TO EAT AND TRAVEL SAFELY

1. "Gluten-free Diet Appeals to 30 Percent of Adults, Survey Says," Huffington Post, www.huffingtonpost.com, March 6, 2013.

CHAPTER 12. SOCIALIZING

1. T. A. Kabbani et al., "Patients with Celiac Disease Have a Lower Prevalence of Non-Insulin-Dependent Diabetes Mellitus and Metabolic Syndrome," *Gastroenterology* 144, no. 5 (May 2013): 912–17.e1.

2. Ibid.

3. Ibid.

CHAPTER 13. FRIENDSHIP, DATING, LOVE & SEX

1. C. Ciacci et al., "Sexual Behaviour in Untreated and Treated Coeliac Patients," *European Journal of Gastroenterology & Hepatology* (August 1998): 649–51.

2. Ibid.

Resources

PATIENT MEDICAL SUPPORT WEBSITES

These websites are great sources of medical and lifestyle information.

Beth Israel Deaconess Medical Center, bidmc.org and celiacnow.org
Boston Children's Hospital, childrenshospital.org
Center for Celiac Research & Treatment at Mass General Hospital, celiaccenter
.org
Celiac Disease Center at Columbia University Medical Center, celiacdisease
center.columbia.edu
Children's Gastroenterology Specialists, S.C., kidstummydoc.com
Children's National Medical Center, Washington, DC, childrensnational.org
Connecticut Children's Medical Center, connecticutchildrens.org
Nationwide Children's Hospital in Columbus, OH, nationwidechildrens.org
Stanford Hospital Celiac Sprue Clinic, stanfordhospital.org
Stony Brook Children's Hospital, Stony Brook, NY, stonybrookchildrens.org
The Children's Hospital of Philadelphia, chop.edu
University of California San Diego, Wm. K. Warren Medical Research Center for
Celiac Disease, celiaccenter.ucsd.edu
University of Chicago Celiac Disease Center, cureceliacdisease.org

NATIONAL SUPPORT GROUP ORGANIZATIONS

These groups have invaluable information on diet and diagnosis as well as links
to local chapters.

Celiac Disease Foundation (CDF), celiac.org

Celiac Support Association (CSA) (formerly Celiac Sprue Association), csaceliacs
.info

Gluten Intolerance Group of North America (GIG), www.gluten.net

REGIONAL SUPPORT GROUP ORGANIZATIONS

Celiac Community Foundation of Northern California, celiaccommunity.org

New England Celiac Organization (NECO) formerly The Healthy Villi, www
.neceliac.org

Westchester Celiac Sprue Support Group, westchesterceliacs.org

INFORMATION, ADVOCACY, AND AWARENESS

American Celiac Disease Alliance (ACDA), americanceliac.org

Clinical Guidelines: Diagnosis and Management of Celiac Disease, American
College of Gastroenterology, gi.org (clinical guidelines)

Food Allergy Research and Education (FARE), foodallergy.org

Food Allergy Research & Resource Program (FARRP), farrp.unl.edu

National Digestive Diseases Information Clearinghouse (NDDIC), digestive.niddk
.nih.gov

National Foundation for Celiac Awareness (NFCA), celiaccentral.org

National Institutes of Health (NIH) Celiac Disease Awareness Campaign, celiac
.nih.gov

National Library of Medicine (NLM), nlm.nih.gov/medlineplus/celiacdisease.html

MORE INFORMATION

On Breastfeeding and Introducing Gluten to Infants

"Breastfeeding and the Use of Human Milk," policy statement from the American Academy of Pediatrics Policy

"Prevalence of Childhood Celiac Disease and Changes in Infant Feeding," by
A. Ivarsson, *Pediatrics*, February 18, 2013

"Who Has the Guts for Gluten?" by Moises Velasquez-Manoff, *New York Times*,
February 23, 2013

On Seniors and Celiac Disease

"When CD Comes with Age," by Mary Beth Schweigert, *Gluten-free Living*, June
2013

GenCare Lifestyle, gencarelifestyle.com; www.gluten.net

On Gluten Ataxia

"Spectrum of Gluten-Related Disorders: Consensus on New Nomenclature and Classification," by A. Sapone et al., *BMCMedicine*, February 7, 2012, www.biomedcentral.com

"Dietary Treatment of Gluten Ataxia," by Dr. M. Hadjivassiliou, *Journal of Neurology, Neurosurgery, with Practical Neurology*, February 2003

"Celiac Disease and Gluten Sensitivity," a special health report from *Living Without* magazine, 2013

On the Low-FODMAP Diet

"FODMAP: A Road Map for IBS," by Rory Jones, *Living Without*, February/March 2013

The Complete Low-FODMAP Diet: A Revolutionary Plan for Managing IBS and Other Digestive Disorders, by Sue Shepherd, PhD, Peter Gibson, MD, and William D. Chey, MD

The Low-FODMAP Diet Cookbook: 150 Simple, Flavorful, Gut-Friendly Recipes to Ease the Symptoms of IBS, Celiac Disease, Crohn's Disease, Ulcerative Colitis, and Other Digestive Disorders, by Sue Shepherd, PhD

MORE INFORMATION ABOUT GENETIC TESTS FOR CELIAC DISEASE

cureceliacdisease.org (search genetic testing)

SAMPLE 504 PLANS FOR SCHOOL LUNCHES AND CLASSROOM MANAGEMENT

American Celiac Disease Alliance, americanceliac.org
National Foundation for Celiac Awareness, celiaccentral.org

ONLINE REFERENCES

Celiac.com
Celiacdisease.about.com
Celiac Listserv, CELIAC-subscribe-request@LISTSERV.ICORS.ORG (to subscribe)
PubMed.com (Abstracts of Medical Papers)

Just for Kids

Kid Start Wellness, San Diego support group, kidstartwellness.org
Raising our Celiac Kids (ROCK) (search for ROCK and the geographic area)

Label Systems

Kfk-enjoy.com
Kidcals.com

GLUTEN-FREE DRUG RESOURCES

Sources of Inactive Ingredients

Daily Med, DailyMed.nlm.nih.gov

Medications

Physicians Desk Reference, drugs.com/pdr

OTC and Prescription Medications

Glutenfreedrugs.com

LIFESTYLE PUBLICATIONS

Allergic Living, allergicliving.com
Delight Gluten-free, delightglutenfree.com
Gluten Free & More, glutenfreeandmore.com (formerly *Living Without*)
Gluten Free Living, glutenfreeliving.com
Simply Gluten-free, simplygluten-free.com

RESOURCE BOOKS

These resource books provide essential information on diet, diagnosis, shopping, and lifestyle.

Celiac Disease: A Hidden Epidemic, Revised and Updated Edition, by Peter H. R. Green, MD, and Rory Jones
Celiac Disease and Gluten Sensitivity: A Special Report, by the editors of *Living Without* magazine

The Essential Gluten-free Restaurant Guide, by triumphdining.com
Gluten-free Diet: A Comprehensive Resource Guide, by Shelley Case, RD
Gluten-free Grocery Shopping Guide, by Dainis Matison and Dr. Mara Matison, ceceliasmarketplace.com
The Gluten-free Nutrition Guide, by Tricia Thompson, RD
Let's Eat Out Around the World Gluten Free & Allergy Free, by Kim Koeller. glutenfreepassport.com
Real Life with Celiac Disease, by Melinda Dennis, RD, and Daniel Leffler, MD, MS

COOKBOOKS

Here are some cookbooks from seasoned veterans that will help novices and experts alike.

Cooking for Your Gluten-Free Teen, by Carlyn Berghoff, Sarah Berghoff McClure, Suzanne P. Nelson, and Nancy Ross Ryan
Fast & Simple Gluten-Free, by Gretchen F. Brown, RD
Gluten-Free Baking, by Rebecca Reilly
Gluten-Free Baking Classics, by Annalise Roberts
Gluten-Free Baking for the Holidays, by Jeanne Sauvage
Gluten Free Every Day, by Robert Landolphi
Gluten-Free Makeovers, by Beth Hillson
Gluten-Free 101: Easy, Basic Dishes Without Wheat, by Carol Fenster
Gluten-Free on a Shoestring Breaks Bread, by Nicole Hunn
Great Gluten-Free Vegan Eats, by Allyson Kramer
Nosh on This (gluten-free baking), by Lisa Stander Horel
1,000 Gluten-Free Recipes, by Carol Fenster
Quick-Fix Gluten Free, by Robert Landolphi

LEADING DOCTORS SPECIALIZING IN CELIAC DISEASE (SOME ALSO SPECIALIZE IN GLUTEN SENSITIVITY)

Adult GI

Nielsen Fernandez-Becker, MD (associate director, Celiac Management Clinic at Stanford Hospital)
Sheila Crowe, MD (University of California, San Diego)
Alessio Fasano, MD (Center for Celiac Research at MassGeneral Hospital for Children, Boston, MA)

Z. Myron Falchuck, MD (Beth Israel Deaconess Medical Center, Boston, MA)

Peter H. R. Green, MD (director, Celiac Disease Center at Columbia University Medical Center–New York)

Martin F. Kagnoff, MD (University of California, San Diego)

Ciaran Kelly, MD (Beth Israel Deaconess Medical Center, Boston, MA)

Benjamin Lebwohl, MD (Celiac Disease Center at Columbia University Medical Center–New York)

Daniel Leffler, MD, MS (Beth Israel Deaconess Medical Center, Boston, MA)

Suzanne K. Lewis, MD (Celiac Disease Center at Columbia University Medical Center–New York)

Joseph A. Murray, MD, additional expertise in refractory sprue (Mayo Clinic, Rochester, MN)

Cynthia S. Rudert, MD (Atlanta, GA)

Michael Schuffler, MD (Seattle, WA)

John J. Zone, MD, dermatologist with expertise in dermatitis herpetiformis (University of Utah, Salt Lake City)

Pediatric GI

Amy R. DeFelice, MD (Celiac Disease Center at Columbia University Medical Center–New York)

Alessio Fasano, MD (Center for Celiac Research at MassGeneral Hospital for Children, Boston, MA)

Rose Graham, MD (Mission Children's Hospital, Asheville, NC)

Stefano Guandalini, MD (University of Chicago Celiac Disease Center, Chicago, IL)

Ivor Hill, MD (Nationwide Children's Hospital, Columbus, OH)

Edward Hoffenberg, MD, additional expertise in type 1 diabetes (Children's Hospital, Denver, Denver, CO)

Philip G. Kazlow, MD (Celiac Disease Center at Columbia University Medical Center–New York)

Alan M. Leichtner, MD (Boston Children's Hospital, Boston, MA)

Michelle Pietzak, MD (Los Angeles, CA)

Norelle Rizkalla Reilly, MD (Celiac Disease Center at Columbia University Medical Center–New York)

Registered Dietitians Specializing in Celiac Disease and the GFD

National Association: Academy of Nutrition and Dietetics, Eatright.org

Rachel Begun, MS, RD, CDN, rachelbegun.com/blog

Shelley Case, B.Sc., RD (Saskatchewan, Canada), glutenfreediet.ca
Melinda Dennis, MS, RD, LDN (Beth Israel Deaconess Medical Center, Boston,
    MA), deletethewheat.com
Nancy Patin Falini, MA, RD, LDN (West Chester, PA)
Laurie Higgins, RD (Boston Children's Hospital)
Cynthia Kupper, RD, executive director of GIG, www.gluten.net
Ann Roland Lee, EdD, RD (New York City)
Mary K. Sharrett, MS, RD (Columbus, OH)
Suzanne Simpson, RD (Celiac Disease Center at Columbia University Medical
    Center–New York)
Laurie B. Steenwyk, M.Ed., RD, LDN (Hendersonville, NC)
Tricia Thompson, MS, RD, glutenfreedietian.com

Naturopathic Physicians

National Association: American Association of Naturopathic Physicians,
    naturopathic.org
Christine Doherty, ND, Balance Point Natural Medicine, pointnatural.com
Dr. Jean Layton, ND, "The Gluten-free Doctor," glutenfreedoctor.com; layton
    healthclinic.com
Tom O'Bryan, DC, thedr.com; theglutensummit.com
Dr. Stephen Wangen, ND, IBS Treatment Center, ibstreatmentcenter.com

RESTAURANTS

Online Resources to Help Locate GF-Friendly Restaurants

Celiacrestaurantguide.com (includes Canada and United States; great for chains)
Dineglutenfree.com (app for IPhone and Android)
Glutenfreefun.com
Glutenfreeglobetrotter.com
Glutenfreepassport.com (great for ethnic dining information and international
    travel. Apps, too.)
Glutenfreeregistry.com
Glutenfreetravelsite.com
Glutensniper.com (App for Android)
www.gluten.net (formerly the Gluten-free Restaurant Awareness Program)
Opentable.com (In metropolitan areas; enter the city, "gluten-free," and "open
    table" in the same search box.)

Triumphdining.com (Restaurant and product guides as well as restaurant cards in many languages. Apps, too.)

Urbanspoon.com (Use filter for specific city or area.)

Restaurant Apps

Gluten-free Fast Food

Find Me Gluten Free

I Eat Out Gluten and Allergen Free

Is That Gluten Free (Eating Out)

National Chain Restaurants, Fast Food Establishments, and Some Regional Eateries

One of the most stressful parts about eating out is trying to figure out where to eat safely. Let these national (or regional) chains of restaurants be your beacon to safe, gluten-free friendly food whether you are dining locally or traveling. They all have gluten-free menus and some degree of protocol in the kitchen. As always, confirm that you are being served the gluten-free version. Delegating your diet to a server without checking might result in being gluten-ed by proxy.

FAST-FOOD SPOTS

Arby's	Jamba Juice
Au Bon Pain	Jason's Deli
Boston Market	Panera Bread
Chick-Fil-A	Pei Wei Asian Diner
Cold Stone Creamery	Qdoba Mexican Grill
Così	SaladWorks
Dairy Queen	Sonic
Erbert and Gerbert's Sandwich Shop	TCBY Frozen Yogurt
Jack in the Box	Wendy's

Note: Most fast-food eateries have charts that list the allergens in their foods, but few have established a protocol to safeguard against cross-contamination. The good news is that you can watch your food being prepared and steer clear of obvious pitfalls. The bad news is that lots of meals are being prepared in the same small space.

SIT-DOWN MEALS

Abuelo's
Applebee's
Austin Grill (Washington, DC, area)
Baja Fresh
Bertucci's Italian Restaurant
Biaggi's Ristorante Italiano
BJ's Restaurant & Brewhouse
Bonefish Grill
BR Guest Hospitality Group (brguest hospitality.com, New York City, Florida, Atlantic City, Las Vegas)
Burton's Grill (East Coast)
California Pizza Kitchen
Carrabba's Italian Grill
Chart House
Cheeseburger in Paradise
Chili's
Chipotle Mexican Grill
Chevys Fresh Mex
Chuck E. Cheese's
Claim Jumper
Dave & Busters
Denny's
Donatos
Elephant Walk (Boston area)
Fleming's Prime Steakhouse & Wine Bar
Fresh Brothers (California)
Hooters
Joe's American Bar & Grill (Eastern Massachusetts and Rhode Island)
Legal Sea Foods (East Coast)
Lettuce Entertain You (restaurant chains within this group have gluten-free menus)
LongHorn Steakhouse
Maggiano's Little Italy
Max and Erma's
Max Restaurant Group (Connecticut; Springfield, MA)
Mellow Mushroom
Moe's Southwest Grill
Ninety Nine Restaurant
Not Your Average Joe's
O'Charley's
The Old Spaghetti Factory
Olive Garden
On the Border Mexican Grill & Cantina
Outback Steakhouse
P.F. Chang China Bistro
Pizza Pie Café
Red Lobster
Red Robin
Romano's Macaroni Grill
Ruby Tuesday
Sam & Louie's Neighborhood Restaurant and Pizzeria
Ted's Montana Grill
Texas de Brazil
Uno's Chicago Grill
Wildfire Restaurants (Washington, DC, and Maryland)
Wood-N-Tap (Connecticut)

Restaurant Cards Translated into Several Languages

Allergypassport.com
Brokerfish.com/food-allergy -translation-cards
Glutenfreeglobetrotter.com
Glutenfreepassport.com
Glutenfreetraveler.com
Glutenfreetravelsite.com
Triumphdining.com

GLUTEN-FREE-FRIENDLY COLLEGES

These schools have been given high marks by students and recent graduates. That's not to say that many other schools don't make the grade, too. But this is a good place to begin the college search.

Bard College, Annandale-on-Hudson, New York
Baylor University, Waco, Texas
Carleton College, Northfield, Minnesota
Clark University, Worcester, Massachusetts
Columbia University, New York, New York
Emory University, Atlanta, Georgia
Geneseo College, Geneseo, New York
Georgetown University, Washington, DC
Iowa State University, Ames, Iowa
Ithaca College, Ithaca, New York
Lesley University, Cambridge, Massachusetts
Oregon State University, Corvallis, Oregon
Penn State, State College, Pennsylvania
Southern Methodist University, Dallas, Texas
SUNY Potsdam, Potsdam, New York
Texas A & M Corpus Christi, Corpus Christi, Texas
Tufts University, Medford, Massachusetts
University of Arizona, Tucson, Arizona
University of Colorado Boulder, Boulder, Colorado
University of Connecticut, Storrs, Connecticut
University of New Hampshire, Durham, New Hampshire
University of Notre Dame, Notre Dame, Indiana
University of Tennessee, Knoxville, Tennessee
University of Wisconsin, Madison, Wisconsin
Vanderbilt University, Nashville, Tennessee
Yale University, New Haven, Connecticut

For the most up-to-date lists of colleges, visit celiac.com, glutenfreetravelsite.com (gluten-free college reviews), and udisglutenfree.com. Other resources include:

Online handbooks for college-bound kids, celiaccentral.org
Celiacs and College: Tips for Parents and Prospective Students
Gluten Free Guide to College
Gluten-free Guide to College Living

RESOURCES FOR THE TWENTY-SOMETHING

These bloggers offer a host of information on gluten-free lifestyle, restaurants, products, and personal encounters aimed at gluten-free singles and the twenty-something crowd.

Ccglutenfreed.com
Celiacinthecity.com
Celiac-scoop.com
Celiacsisters.net
Celiacteen.com
Gfreelaura.com
Glutendude.com
Glutenfreebetsy.com
Glutenfreefun.com

Glutenfreegimmethree.com
Glutenfreeglobetrotter.com,
Gluten-free.meetup.com; see also
    Gluten-free MeetUp New York
Glutenfreesingles.com
Glutenfreeways.com
Singleswithfoodallergies.com
Sprinklesandallergies.com
Youngwildandgfree.com

GROCERY SHOPPING

Online Shopping

There's a plethora of gluten-free products available on market shelves. Nevertheless, for those hard-to-find items, mail order may be the best bet. Check out these websites.

Amazon.com
Bobsredmill.com
Food4Celiacs.com (Gluten-free
    Trading Company)
Freefromgluten.com
GlutenFreeMall.com

GlutenFreeSmartStore.com
GlutenFreePalace.com
Glutino.com
Kingarthurflour.com/glutenfree/
Kinnikinnick.com
Quattrobimbi.com

Shopping Guides

Essential Gluten-free Grocery Guide,
    triumphdining.com

Gfreek.com (product and service reviews)
Gluten-free Grocery Shopping Guide

Apps for Shopping

Fooducate for Allergies
Is That Gluten Free?

ipiit, The Food Ambassador (food and
    ingredient information)

STOCKING YOUR GLUTEN-FREE PANTRY

The products here are gluten free but not every product from every company is safe for your diet. This list is by no means exhaustive, but it gives you a good place to start.

Asian Sauces (including curry pastes, tamari sauce, fish sauce, and stir-fry sauces)

San-J
Thai Kitchen
Wok Mei

Baking Mixes (cake, muffin, bread, piecrust, pancake, and cookie mixes)

Bella Gluten-free
Betty Crocker
Bob's Red Mill
Breads by Anna
Chebe
Glutino Gluten-free Pantry
Jules Gluten Free
King Arthur
Kinnikinnick
Mina's
Moon Rabbit Mixes
Namaste Foods
1-2-3 Gluten Free
Orgran
Pamela's Products
Tom Sawyer All-Purpose Blend

Bread Crumbs

Aleia's
Dr. Schär
Glutino
Ian's
Kinnikinnick

Breads

Against the Grain
Canyon Bakehouse
Dr. Schär
Glutino
Kinnikinnick
Orgran
Rudi's
Three Bakers
Udi's

Canned Chili

Amy's Vegetarian Chili
Hormel Chili *with* Beans
Shelton Turkey Chili

Chicken Broth

Kitchen Basics
Progresso
Swanson brand (check labels)

Chicken Nuggets

Applegate Naturals
Bell & Evans
Ian's
Perdue Simply Smart
Tyson

Chocolate Sauce

Ah! Laska
Hershey's
Smuckers

Cold Cuts
Applegate Farms
Boar's Head
Dietz & Watson
Jennie-O
Jones Dairy Farm
Niman Ranch
Oscar Mayer
Wellshire Farms

Corn Tortillas
Mission Foods
La Tortilla Factory

Cookies
Dr. Schär
Enjoy Life Foods
Glutino
Kinnikinnick
Mi-Del
Pamela's Products
Udi's

Crackers
Crunchmaster
Dr. Schär
Glutino
Kinnikinnick
Orgran

Croutons
Gillian's Foods
Glutino
Olivia's Croutons

Crushed Garlic and Chopped Basil (freezer section)
Dorot brand

Doughnuts
Kinnikinnick

Flours
Ancient Harvest (quinoa)
Authentic Foods
The Birkett Mills (buckwheat)
Bob's Red Mill
Château Cream Hill Estates (oats)
GF Harvest
Gluten-free Oats (oats)
Montana Gluten Free

Flour Wraps
French Meadow
La Tortilla Factory (teff wraps)
Rudi's
Toufayan
Udi's

Ice Cream and Frozen Yogurt (check labels as a few flavors contain wheat or barley)
Ben and Jerry's
Edy's
Häagen-Daz
Hood
Judy's Gluten-free Ice Cream Sandwiches
So Delicious (dairy-free, too)
Turkey Hill

Pasta

Ancient Harvest (with quinoa)
Barilla
DeBoles
DeLallo
Jovial
Le Veneziane
Ronzoni
Sam Mills
Tinkyada
truRoots (Ancient Grains)

Pizza Crusts

Amy's Kitchen
Bold
Dr. Schär
Ener-G
Glutino
French Meadow
Ian's
JD's
Kinnikinnick
Orgran
Pillsbury (refrigerated dough)
Venice Pizza
Udi's

Pizza Sauce

Muir Glen
Ragú

Soups and Broths

Amy's
Imagine Foods
Pacific
Progresso
Shelton
Wolfgang Puck

Toaster Pastries

Glutino

Yogurt

Note that most plain yogurt is safe.
Avoid yogurt with crunch toppings.

Activia
Brown Cow
Cabot
Chobani
Dannon
Fage
Nogurt (dairy-free)
So Delicious (dairy-free)
Stonyfield Farms
WholeSoy & Co (dairy-free)
Yoplait

VITAMINS AND SUPPLEMENTS

Here's a partial list of companies that manufacture gluten-free dietary supplements.

Country Life
Dr. Doherty's, glutenfreevitamins.com
Enzymedica

Freeda Vitamins
Nature's Bounty
Pioneer Nutritional Formulas

Kids' Vitamins

CVS Brand Animal Shapes
Li'l Critter
Nature's Plus
Nordic Berries
Organic Yummi Bears

Calcium Supplements

Caltrate
Citracal
Country Life
Viactive

More on Supplements

"Nutrient Know-How," by Eve Becker, *Living Without* magazine, April/May 2014

BREAD MACHINES FOR GLUTEN-FREE BREAD

Many bread machines are suitable for making gluten-free bread. They come in a wide range of prices and features. Look for a machine that has a gluten-free cycle, a programmable cycle, or both. If you don't eat a lot of bread, select a machine that makes a one-pound loaf. If you go through a lot of bread, pick one that is best for a 1½- to 2-pound loaf.

Breadman
Breville
Cuisinart
Hamilton Beach
Oster

Panasonic
Sunbeam
T-Fal
West Bend
Zojirushi

TOAST-IT REUSABLE TOASTER BAGS

Amazon.com
Vat19.com

CAMPING FOODS THAT DO DOUBLE DUTY

Several companies specialize in camping and on-the-go shelf stable gluten-free foods. They are perfect for survival kits, too.

Alpineairefoods.com
Augasonfarms.com
Bakeryonmain.com
Glutenfreeemergencykits.com

Gonealpine.com
Gopicnic.com
Lovegrownfoods.com
Preparewise.com

ONLINE MONEY-SAVER SITES

These websites are just a few that offer everything from Groupon-style savings to discount coupons.

Abesmarket.com

Amazon.com

Befreeforme.com

Glutenfreecoupons.com

Glutenfreedeals.com

Glutenfreemall.com

GlutenFreeSaver.com

Vitacost.com (vitamins, gluten-free
products and great coupons)

Metric Conversions

The recipes in this book have not been tested with metric measurements, so some variations might occur.

Remember that the weight of dry ingredients varies according to the volume or density factor: 1 cup of flour weighs far less than 1 cup of sugar, and 1 tablespoon doesn't necessarily hold 3 teaspoons.

General Formula for Metric Conversion

Ounces to grams . . . . . Multiply ounces by 28.35
Grams to ounces . . . . . Multiply grams by 0.035
Pounds to grams . . . . . Multiply pounds by 453.5
Pounds to kilograms . . Multiply pounds by 0.45
Cups to liters . . . . Multiply cups by 0.24
Fahrenheit to Celsius . . Subtract 32 from Fahrenheit temperature, multiply by 5, divide by 9
Celsius to Fahrenheit . . Multiply Celsius temperature by 9, divide by 5, add 32

Weight (Mass) Measurements

1 ounce = 30 grams
2 ounces = 55 grams
3 ounces = 85 grams
4 ounces = ¼ pound = 125 grams
8 ounces = ½ pound = 240 grams
12 ounces = ¾ pound = 375 grams
16 ounces = 1 pound = 454 grams

Volume (Dry) Measurements

¼ teaspoon = 1 milliliter
½ teaspoon = 2 milliliters
¾ teaspoon = 4 milliliters
1 teaspoon = 5 milliliters
1 tablespoon = 15 milliliters
¼ cup = 59 milliliters
⅓ cup = 79 milliliters
½ cup = 118 milliliters
⅔ cup = 158 milliliters
¾ cup = 177 milliliters
1 cup = 225 milliliters
4 cups or 1 quart = 1 liter
½ gallon = 2 liters
1 gallon = 4 liters

Linear Measure

½ inch = 1½ cm
1 inch = 2½ cm
6 inches = 15 cm
8 inches = 20 cm
10 inches = 25 cm
12 inches = 30 cm
20 inches = 50 cm

Volume (Liquid) Measurements

1 teaspoon = ⅙ fluid ounce = 5 milliliters
1 tablespoon = ½ fluid ounce = 15 milliliters
2 tablespoons = 1 fluid ounce = 30 milliliters
¼ cup = 2 fluid ounces = 60 milliliters
⅓ cup = 2⅔ fluid ounces = 79 milliliters
½ cup = 4 fluid ounces = 118 milliliters
1 cup or ½ pint = 8 fluid ounces = 250 milliliters
2 cups or 1 pint = 16 fluid ounces = 500 milliliters
4 cups or 1 quart = 32 fluid ounces = 1,000 milliliters
1 gallon = 4 liters

Oven Temperature Equivalents
Fahrenheit (F) and Celsius (C)

100°F = 38°C
200°F = 95°C
250°F = 120°C
300°F = 150°C
350°F = 180°C
400°F = 205°C
450°F = 230°C

Acknowledgments

In "Friends Don't Let Friends Eat Gluten," I talk about the importance of creating a support network. I am grateful to mine for lending their expertise and time to this project.

Among them, heartfelt thanks go to Robert G. Schwartz, MD. Like my family, he lives a multidimensional gluten-free life as a celiac patient, a gastroenterologist, and the parent of a daughter with celiac disease. I am indebted to Bob for his insights, both personal and professional.

I am also indebted to Andrea Levario, JD, executive director of the American Celiac Disease Alliance, who read this manuscript with an expertise that comes from years of advocating for patients and working with all aspects of this field. Andrea is also the parent of a child with celiac disease, Pablo, who I met when he was three. Now in high school, Pablo is thriving gluten-free.

A huge thanks to Alice Bast, president of the National Foundation for Celiac Awareness (NFCA), Nancy Ginter, director of operations, and Jennifer North, vice president, at NFCA, who provided a wealth of information that helped me frame this book.

Heartfelt thanks go to the following who I turned to for fact checking, quotes, and advice: Erin Smith, Gluten-free MeetUp New York; Lindsey Schnitt, youngwildandgfree.com; Stefano Guandalini, MD, founder and medical director, University of Chicago Celiac Disease Center; Peter H. R. Green, MD, director, Celiac Disease Center, Columbia University; Kelsey

Haggett; Joseph A. Murray, MD, clinical practitioner and researcher, Department of Gastroenterology and Hepatology, Mayo Clinic, Rochester, MN; Rory Jones, coauthor, *Celiac Disease: A Hidden Epidemic*; Lauren Komack, MSW; Robert Landolphi, culinary operations manager, Dining Services, University of Connecticut and glutenfreechef.com; Sybil Nassau, branch manager, Gluten Intolerance Group ShorelineEast, Old Saybrook, CT; Peter Pollay, chef/owner of Posana Café, Asheville, NC; Janet Rinehart, president, Houston Celiac Support Group; Mary Schucklebier, executive director, Celiac Support Association; Tracy Struckrath, Thrive! Meetings and Events; and Lisa Walton, codirector, Camp Celiac. A heartfelt thanks also goes to Cynthia Kupper, RD, executive director, and Channon Quinn, director, Industry Division, Gluten Intolerance Group of North America; Christine Doherty, ND, Balance Point Natural Medicine; Steve Plogsted, PharmD, clinical pharmacist, Nationwide Childrens Hospital, Columbus, OH, and glutenfreedrugs.com; Deborah Ceizler, chief development officer, Celiac Disease Foundation; and Steve Taylor, PhD, codirector, Food Allergy Research and Resource Program (FARRP).

I am indebted to several people who helped turn this concept into a book. It's an understatement to say I could not do this without them. Gratitude to my talented agents, good friends, and compatriots on the special diet highway, Sally and Lisa Ekus, and to my amazing editor, Renée Sedliar, who made this book a reality. I am grateful for her vision and her detail. I am also thankful for Claire Ivett at Perseus Books, who lent an extra pair of eyes to this project. I'd be remiss if I didn't acknowledge Cisca Schreefel and the diligent copyeditors at Da Capo. They are the icing on this gluten-free cake.

Thanks to Laura Kuykendall, Sophie Gardner, Patrick Bernard, and the whole team at Glutino and to my colleagues at Gluten Free and More— Eve Becker, Tom Canfield, Oksana Charla, Tim Cole, Robert Englander, Laurel Greene, Phil Penny, Madalene Rhyand, and Alicia Woodward.

Finally, gratitude and hugs to my son, Jeremy, for endless life experiences including the privilege of raising a child with celiac disease; to my sister, Jennifer, who has served as a guinea pig for my culinary experiments and experiential stories; and to my husband, Joel, my fellow traveler on this gluten-free journey.

Index